HELP YOURSELF HEAL

HELP YOURSELF HEAL

8 STEPS TO HEALTH & WHOLENESS

BILL L. LITTLE, Ph.D.

CompCare® Publishers

2415 Annapolis Lane
Minneapolis, Minnesota 55441

Little, Bill L., 1935-
    Help yourself heal / by Bill L. Little.
        p. 118 cm.
    "8 steps to health & wholeness based on a clinical study on cancer
and longevity"—Cover.
    Includes bibliographical references.
    ISBN 0-89638-200-1: $7.95
    1. Cancer—Alternative treatment.   2. Holistic medicine.
3. Mental healing.   4. Visualization.   I. Title.
RC271.A62L57   1990
962.1'96994—dc20   89-25386
                                                              CIP

Cover and interior design by Nancy MacLean

    Inquiries, orders, and catalog requests should be addressed to
    CompCare Publishers
    2415 Annapolis Lane
    Minneapolis, MN 55441
    Call toll free 800/328-3330
    (Minnesota residents 612/559-4800)

5   4   3   2   1
94   93   92   91   90

To my parents, E. T. Little and Beulah Dile,
and to my grandchildren,
Candace and Shaun Schnurbusch,
and Tyler Butler

Acknowledgments

I am grateful to many people for helping make this book possible. If there are omissions in this list of acknowledgments, they are entirely unintentional.

Thanks to my friends Royal Eaton, M.D.; Juan Cardin, M.D.; Carlos Perez, M.D.; Lily Hanes, M.D.; Robert Baglan, M.D.; Darrell Pitt, D.O.; and many others in the medical community who helped me with information, guidance, and the referral of patients.

A special word of thanks goes to the cancer patients who have encouraged me in this writing. Among those who have worked hard for their own health and taught me so very much are David Kendall, Judy Hunt, Jan Bolger, Lou Fine, John Metz, Vita Epiphanio, Maxine Bruegge, and many others. Some wonderful people, who also worked with me and from whom I have drawn inspiration, are among those who fought gallantly for life but have not survived. They include Clint Rayford, Judy Bean, Don Niggeman, and Walter Grueninger.

I, and every person who may be helped by this book, also owe a debt of gratitude to my good friend and co-worker Gay Carlstrom. She not only worked diligently on the manuscript and offered many helpful suggestions, but if she had not encouraged me to proceed—and even at times insisted—I probably would not have written this book.

Thanks to editors Jane Thomas Noland and Jane Thomas for their suggestions and patience.

I also thank the people of Christ Memorial Baptist Church, my wife, Yvonne, and my family for their support.

• CONTENTS •

Introduction

This book is long overdue and I am pleased that my friend Bill Little has finally decided to write it. I have had the opportunity to observe the effectiveness of the techniques Bill uses.

The material contained within is a practical, simple, and effective guide to adjunctive cancer therapy.

As a pulmonary physician, I see too many patients with lung cancer. When told the diagnosis, they almost always ask, "How long do I have to live?"

The truth is, no one knows how long anyone has to live. Doctors don't know everything. In fact, some doctors don't seem to know anything! There are people walking around now who think they're healthy who will be dead before the most recently diagnosed cancer patient.

We frequently see patients with far advanced cancer who live much longer than expected. We also see patients with controllable disease who succumb rapidly. The differences I'm sure spring from the mental and emotional resources of the patient.

Nurses frequently note, "It's too bad he died. He was such a nice guy." I believe that in this case nice guys are finished first. Some people are natural victims. Survivors are curmudgeons who ask questions, and disagree when they need to. They take responsibility for their illness. They choose to live longer. This book can help people choose life.

We read in the tabloids about celebrities who are "battling cancer." Are they really, or are they acquiescing, passive victims?

People with cancer, or indeed any illness, must take responsibility for their care. In our pulmonary rehabilitation program, exercise is a vital component. Those who do the prescribed exercises get better. Those who want to get everything from a pill don't get better.

Rats inoculated with cancer cells, then exposed to the stress of random electric shocks all developed cancer and died from it, whereas only half the control rats developed cancer and lived twice as long before death.

Objective studies show diminished cellular immunity in people under stress, which recovers when the stress is removed. Tumor "search and destroy" missions in the body are conducted by the cellular immunity.

If stress can contribute to the cause of cancer, it seems reasonable to many of us that reducing stress can ameliorate its effects. Dr. Little's work confirms this to be the case.

One in every 800,000 cases of cancer undergoes spontaneous remission. We don't know why. Miracle? Chance? Act of God? Is it possibly a change in that person's immune system? Is it possible that the person started doing something right, such as reducing stress?

The precepts in this book are important. You should question your doctors. You have a right to. It is your body. People are afraid of asking a stupid question. The only stupid question is the one you didn't ask when you needed an answer. Take responsibility for your illness. No one else will care as much about the result as you do.

Valuable as this book will be for cancer patients, its usefulness is not limited to them. The techniques described—relaxation, imagery, visualization, and cognitive restructing—are applicable to most of us.

Preventive measures are potentially more important than therapeutic ones. I am convinced that every illness known to man, from chillblains to hangnail, is worse if you are anxious, worried, or upset. I would not hesitate to recommend this book to people who are anxious, depressed, or just plain worried.

Dr. Little has not written a Pollyanna guide. The techniques are described in practical and useful detail.

If you have cancer—or a loved one has cancer—use these techniques as adjuncts to prescribed therapy, surgery, radiation, and chemotherapy. There is no substitute for doing all you can to help yourself. Even if an individual's life is not prolonged, the quality of a life with reduced stress must be enhanced.

There is quiet wisdom in this book. Use it. No matter how well you believe you're doing, why not take a chance on doing better?

Royal J. Eaton, M.D., F.C.C.P.
Consultant in pulmonary medicine for Christian
Hospitals, Northeast and Northwest, St. Louis;
Assistant professor, Washington University
School of Medicine

Please Read This First

I sincerely wish that everyone would read this book or one like it or would at least get to know the basic facts and theories presented here. I'm a realist though, and I know that fewer than 10 per cent of the people who read books will read beyond the second chapter.

I want to share with you the basic measures I recommend to every cancer patient I see. I believe that these practices will help people stay well, prevent disease, and help many of the sick recover.

Since I can't be sure that 90 per cent of you will stick with me and read beyond chapter two, here in the introduction I want to summarize the guidelines that will help you help yourself toward a healthier life.

The first thing I tell people I work with is to make a choice. Do you want to live or die? About two of every five have not yet made that decision. Some decide to die, some to live, but all of them choose. If your life situation is so bad that you want to get out at any price, even the price of death, then you may decide to die. Most people prefer life to the unknown, but are not highly motivated to live. Every day we decide in one way or another to push the live button or the die button. What is your choice today?

I naively thought that cancer patients would do just about anything to get well, just as professional athletes work hard to improve their chances to succeed. I was wrong! I have counseled approximately one hundred cancer patients in the last ten years. Fewer than half of them report that they follow through on the stress reduction, visualization, exercise, and thought-changing programs I recommend. This was true even though every patient I questioned believed that the program would or could help them.

In retrospect, I know that the lack of commitment shouldn't surprise me. Not when people continue smoking in the face of all the negative evidence concerning tobacco and disease. Not when people refuse to change their diets despite their knowledge that different foods would be healthier. And not when even professional athletes do not follow through on programs that have helped them improve their performance.

This knowledge boils down to a fact that is hard to accept. Most of us want someone or something to be responsible for us. We want a doctor, a pill, or God to solve our problems, but we are just not committed to working for ourselves.

There is little doubt that practically all of us *know* better than we *do*; we're wiser in thought than in action. The tragedy is that all the knowledge in the world will not make us more successful or healthier if we lack the discipline to apply what we know.

If your choice is to live and stay healthy, then I suggest that you begin a regular relaxation program. All of us need to make a specific and special effort to incorporate regular times of relaxation in our lives. This conscious planning will become more and more vital in years to come as the pace of living increases and personal life stress rises.

A part of your relaxation program should include deep breathing. Stop what you're doing for a few minutes several times a day, and take about eight to ten breaths. Then relax your muscles in groups by beginning at the top of your head and moving your attention to different muscle groups through your body.

Take time each day to visualize or picture health in your life. See yourself as a healthy person. Visualize yourself relaxing and enjoying life. Play with your imagination. In your mind's eye, you can be anything you want. Imagine that your immune system is powerful and active. See your own white blood cells vigilantly moving through your blood stream looking for invaders. When they find one, they attack. They certainly attack cancer cells and destroy them.

Think about your purpose in life. Make some definite plans. Set some goals for six months, a year, three years, and five years from now. Goals activate us. Purpose generates energy. Good clear goals give us a "why." People certainly live better and probably live longer with goals.

Begin a moderate exercise program. Don't overdo, but do! People are healthier and live longer on the average if they exercise.

Eat better! I don't mean more. Eat less, but eat better foods. Use some common sense. Add fiber to your diet, and eat plenty of fruit, especially early in the day. Be sure you are giving your body good nutrients. Your car will not run without fuel, and neither will your body.

Have fun. Play a little; laugh a little. Determine to enjoy your life as much as you can. Laughter is a stress breaker. Joy energizes. If you laugh more, you'll live more! We need a balance between work and play.

Decide what you believe in. A strong philosophy or strong religious faith can add strength to your system.

Here in a nutshell is a summary of the program that the rest of this book will describe in detail. Knowing what to do and accepting responsibility for doing it are inseparable twins in health. To do without knowing is dangerous. To know without doing is useless. To know and do is healing.

That's it, a summary of the program described in this

book, eight simple principles for good health:

1. Make a conscious choice to live.
2. Relax daily.
3. Use positive visualization.
4. Set goals.
5. Exercise regularly.
6. Eat sensibly.
7. Enjoy life.
8. Believe in something greater than yourself.

A Personal Note

For about twelve years, I have been involved in cancer research at three major Midwest hospitals, believing that I can make a contribution to the treatment and prevention of the disease. Several books have influenced my research. They are among the growing body of literature that links emotions to physical illnesses, particularly cancer. This "new" concept actually goes back at least as far as Galen, a doctor who lived a century or two after Jesus.

I first read a book by Glenn Clark that is no longer in print. It is the remarkably insightful book, *How to Find Health Through Prayer*. Clark suggests that there is a relationship between various diseases and emotional states. Lawrence LeShan supports Clark's ideas in his fascinating study of emotional causation in cancer, *You Can Fight for Your Life*.

These two books offer spiritual and psychological theories. Carl and Stephanie Simonton's handbook, *Getting Well Again*, applies the theories to life in a practical way. And recently the popular book, *Unlimited Power*, by Anthony Robbins has encouraged further looks at psychological state and nutrition, and at the way we talk to ourselves and imagine our lives. Robbins thinks these factors might be important in the cure and prevention of cancer and other diseases.

Love, Medicine and Miracles, by a surgeon, Bernie Siegel, M.D., combines the best ideas in all four of these works and applies them specifically to cancer patients.

Perhaps the most interesting and helpful connections are found in the relationship between stress and disease. Since the extensive research of Hans Seive, the acknowledged expert in the study of stress and its effects on human beings, there has been a growing belief that stress retards the immune system, thus making the body more susceptible to disease. If this is the case, then all diseases, including cancer, are more likely when the body is stressed.

Eventually, I became interested in imagery or visualization, first in connection with cancer patients. Later I used the process to help professional baseball players. Their performance improved, especially the pitchers'.

Imagery is the process by which a person employs imagination to assist the body's natural resources. We may close our eyes and imagine just about anything. I recommend that cancer patients imagine their bodies using their white blood cells to fight cancer cells.

My reading and my personal experience with sick people led me to think for a long time that, if people improved the quality of their lives, they generally lived longer. There were plenty of anecdotes to support the idea. I both heard and read stories about people who fought the odds and lived in spite of "terminal" illnesses. They overcame cancer and other dreaded diseases by changing their life styles. They relaxed, visualized, became more positive, and expressed their feelings. The result? According to the anecdotes, they lived longer.

Twelve years ago, I set out to test my experience with a scientific study. After two years at a local hospital, I moved to a major research hospital, where I did another seven-year study.

The people who agreed to participate in our research were being treated by doctors and nutritionists and other medical specialists. We asked these patients to build a healthier life style on that medical foundation. We found clear evidence that the cancer patients in our group who practiced the program outlined in this book lived longer than those who did not. Also they said that the program gave them more energy and hope and happiness. So they had more life, and their lives were worth living.

We studied only a small number of patients, and our findings need to be tested with more research. But in the meantime, it can't hurt us to live healthier, happier lives while we wait for science to verify the research that has already been done.

We all tend to be lopsided, but we need to remain in balance. We can maintain balance only if we remember our foundations. Some would-be philosophers stare at their navels. It seems to me that we should pay more attention to our feet. Foundations are vital!

I learned the importance of building on foundations when I was in college. I was one of several basketball players who were in an algebra class together. We took the course because it was taught by the assistant athletic director. One fellow knew some algebra; call him LaMar. A second, Don, knew a little bit. The third, Jimmy, knew about as much algebra as the average mailbox.

In one test, Jimmy scored the highest grade. All of us were puzzled as to how this could occur. We asked our coach, who sized up the situation immediately.

He pointed to this logic. "LaMar knew some answers. Don knew some and copied others from LaMar's paper. Jimmy may have known one answer and copied from Don's paper. That means Jimmy had the benefit of what LaMar knew and what Don knew, in addition to the little bit he knew himself."

Jimmy would have been utterly stupid to think that his own limited knowledge was all that he needed. He built on the foundation of others.

Sick people need the same approach from their helpers. Some "experts" believe that their treatment, their own solitary answer, is the only really valid approach. This kind of one-man show sacrifices the powerful benefits of teamwork. If physicians, psychologists, nutritionists, clerics, and other practitioners work together and treat a sick patient as a member of the team, each person builds on the foundation of all the others' efforts. The power of the whole, acting together, is greater than the power of the separate parts, acting in isolation.

People really are whole beings and need to be treated as such.

• ONE •

I Have Stories to Tell

Most medical people I've met care about their patients and are searching for ways to help. Their cups of knowledge are not so full that more cannot be poured into them. Many welcome input from psychology and religion.

None of us has the total answer. The program described in this book is just one of the steps that can help patients of all kinds, especially cancer patients. It can also be used to help prevent disease. The emphasis is on the word "help." As psychology and religion are not the total answer, neither is surgery, nor exercise, nor chemotherapy. We all need to work together hand-in-hand with the patient. Each helper must build on the foundation the others have laid. And all must respect the power of the patient's own inner resources.

I have seen some fantastically encouraging things occur with cancer patients. Two-and-a-half years ago, for example, a man named Dave came into my office. His doctor had diagnosed lung cancer six months earlier, and had removed the upper right lobe of his lung. In December, Dave had been told that the cancer had spread to the stem of his brain.

It was late December when Dave came to see me on a referral by his radiologist. His physician had told him that his life expectancy was short, perhaps three months at most. It was a compassionate thing to tell him, because the tumor in his brain stem would cause pressure, resulting in a coma. He needed to get his legal affairs in order before he became incapacitated. His internist and his oncologist had confirmed the prognosis.

Frankly, Dave looked terrible. He was thin. He wore a wig. His face was drawn. "Why did you make the appointment to see me?" I asked him.

"I know you've worked with cancer patients," he said, "and I'm hoping you can help me deal with this situation."

I knew he was referring to his own death. "You think you are dying?"

"Yes. I need help in facing this," he said.

Dave was obviously resigned and concerned. My own reaction to the prospect of my death would not have been so matter-of-fact, nor spoken so softly and with such control.

"Do you want to work on getting well?" I asked him.

I have learned that people do not answer that question with an automatic "yes." Many patients have decided far in advance of treatment that they are tired of living. Some make this choice consciously, and some unconsciously. Others have a dogged determination to live. Even if the patients are clear in their replies, they sometimes change their minds later on.

Dave answered with surprise, "I didn't know I had a choice!"

"Of course you do." I paused, wanting to remain positive and still maintain integrity. "There are no guarantees, but it can happen. You can get well, and I'm willing to help you any way that I can."

I really meant it, and he knew that. I believe therapists or physicians have better results if they really care about their patients, if they love them. This feeling cannot be faked, but if it is real, the patient's trust grows.

I wanted to feed into his mind every positive thought possible. We certainly have too few of them. I belong to the school that believes in hope. Many of us are accused of giving false hope, but we respond, "There is no such thing as false hope, only hope." If I am to face death, I would rather do it with my heart filled with hope than to face it with despair.

At that moment, we began a restructuring of Dave's every negative thought, the first step in improving his health. This process, called "cognitive restructuring," would consciously change Dave's belief system, his ideas, from weak and negative to strong and positive. (The method is the subject of chapter three, "You Can Change Your Mind.")

Next, we developed skills to help Dave relax. We did this because of all the emphasis on stress and disease. It appears that stress retards our immune systems and makes us more susceptible to all kinds of disease, even cancer. If that is true, it would stand to reason that reducing stress would free our immune systems and give us a better chance to fight cancer and win!

Another set of skills Dave and I started working on has to do with positive imagery. I don't know how or why this technique works, but it does. Somehow our bodies seem to produce or do the things we most clearly picture in our minds. All of us see visions of ourselves in our own imagination continually, every day. People who are obsessed with visions of sickness frequently become ill.

On the other hand, we believe that people who are obsessed with thoughts of wellness get well, or at least have a better chance than those who are focused on disease. All of us could learn from this fact some valuable ideas for better health. It makes sense to me that what helps us get well could prevent our getting sick. So I encourage people to talk, think, and imagine being healthy.

Dave and I also talked about exercise. We worked up a plan that would be reasonable for him. Within days, he joined a health club. Interestingly, he took a three-month membership, which he happily changed later on to a "lifetime" membership.

Then Dave went to a nutritionist, but she unfortunately believed that nutrition is the total solution to all health problems. Doctors aren't the only ones who think they have all the answers. There are many psychologists, sociologists, clergy, and nutritionists with the same problem. Perhaps that is just a human problem. A good rule of thumb is never to trust anyone totally who speaks with the certainty of God. So Dave and I worked together to weed out the nutritionist's grandiosity and salvage her best ideas.

We then talked about Dave's faith in God. Most people have this faith. They are just not clear about it. Clarity of faith brings a sense of security and peace that further reduces stress and frees the body to use its healing system.

Dave worked diligently in all these ways. He became more open about his feelings. He designed more fun into his life. He practiced relaxation and imagery at least three times a day. He changed his internal belief system. He clarified his faith. He improved his diet, adding more fiber with fruits and vegetables, and he exercised regularly.

In three months, Dave was not in a coma. He and his wife were skiing in Aspen, Colorado!

By midsummer they were vacationing in New England. (I got a can of pure maple syrup from that trip.)

A year later, he was fighting a recurrence. He had fluid on his lungs removed and needed massive doses of chemotherapy for a metastasis (spreading) of cancer to his right hip.

The chemo was "supposed" to make him sick. I said, "Don't make book on that."

The morning after massive chemotherapy doses, I asked how he was doing.

He said, "Anyone who had bet I'd be sick would have lost money."

"What are you doing now?" He sounded so chipper, I wondered if he planned on staying home all day.

"My wife, my son, and I are going to see the Blues play hockey tonight," he said.

This answer typifies Dave's reaction to trouble now. Dave consistently responds to treatment better than expected, and together, we are fighting for his life. We believe we can and will win.

The bottom line of the story is still unwritten, but the fact is that Dave believes he would have been dead a year ago if it had not been for his participation in his own health program.

I asked him what the major contribution from our relationship has been and he said, "You have given me hope!" He later added that, along with hope, he had learned things he could do to help himself.

"People stand a better chance of being healthy, getting well, or preventing disease," he says, "if they participate in their own health care, if they help themselves."

Another patient came to my office last January. Ann, a thirty-four-year-old cancer patient, had had a mastectomy; one of her breasts had been removed surgically. Cancer had now involved her lymph system.

She was in a state of total despair and fatigue. If not consciously, she had at least decided unconsciously that she wanted to die.

When I saw her for the second time, I asked her if she was interested in reconstructive surgery. Her response was, "I thought about it, but there's no point to doing it."

I didn't have to ask why. She was not interested in living that long and believed she was dying then.

There are lots of reasons people opt to die. They may find responsibilities too much to endure. They may be unhappy in marriage and unable to divorce. Death is a way out. They may feel guilty about some real or imaginary sin

5

and have no sense of a forgiving God; thus, they think they "deserve" death. They may have failed in some endeavor and feared humiliation. The list goes on!

The fact is that when people decide consciously or unconsciously to die, there is little that can be done for them. My challenge in this case was not only to provide skills with which Ann could participate in her own recovery and treatment. It was to help her face the reality of her choice.

She went through a soul-searching struggle and consciously made the decision to live. She has questioned that decision a few times but still seems clear in her commitment to live as long as she can. She has been examined and is scheduled for reconstructive surgery soon. Her life is presently happier than it has ever been.

She is finding useful activities for herself and is consciously seeking to deepen her religious faith. With the discovery of her worth as an object of God's love, as one with purpose and a right to express her feelings, she has experienced a growing sense of peace and strength.

She is practicing relaxation and imagery. She is exercising. She is watching her diet. She is changing her negative thoughts into more realistic and positive ones. She is growing in personal faith. However long her life may be, she lives with a higher quality of life than she has ever known before. She is living!

There are many other stories. There are happy ones and sad ones. Some people have died, while others have extended their lives, and some are well.

It is hard to judge the meaning for each person. I was disappointed when a fine lady died a few years ago. I said to her oncologist, "I feel like we failed her."

"Failed her? Not by a long shot," he replied. "When we got her, she was dying of lung cancer. Her life expectancy was less than three months."

I remembered the despair she had shown. The

oncologist asked whether I remembered her desire, as well.

Yes, I did.

He continued, as if I didn't remember. "She wanted to live to see her youngest son married the next year and to see her oldest son graduate from one of the Ivy League schools in two years. She saw it all and even the birth of her grandchild. She died happily and peacefully. We did not fail her."

I know he was right. She used all the skills we taught her to live until her goals were reached. Then she died.

When I first met another patient, a jazz drummer named Clint, he weighed 140 pounds and had given up on life. He told me he had rented a room in a local hotel; it was to be the scene of his death.

Again there were many factors involved. He had been through a lot of personal struggles and was tired. Nevertheless, six months later, he weighed 178 pounds and had returned to work, playing jazz drums.

Four years later, Clint and I introduced a video on his approach to jazz drumming.

A year after that, he died peacefully at home, his family intact, his daughter securely in medical school. He and I had also enjoyed five years of remarkable friendship. I mourned his death, but I rejoiced in the five years he said he would not have had without intervention and a change in his attitude.

For whatever reasons, he had stopped the program and all treatment about six months before his death, and he went back into treatment too late to recover. Maybe he had finished his tasks and decided to die. I simply do not know why, but I do know that, both consciously and unconsciously, people make the decision to die.

The list goes on. I remember a patient with Hodgkins disease whose life has been a magnificent example of strength and inspiration for more than ten years now. Vita remains cancer-free, as do many Hodgkins patients, but her story is especially remarkable because Vita is a singer, and radiation had damaged her vocal cords.

Her doctors told her that she'd never be able to sing again. They were wrong! She can "belt" them out with the best of them now. How did she recover? She used relaxation, imagery, and positive attitudes to overcome the damage to her vocal cords.

The methods, techniques, or skills I share with you in this book can help you if you are a cancer patient. You can use these skills to participate in your own health care, as Dave, Ann, Clint, and Vita did.

You can also use these skills to help prevent disease, as well as assist in curing it. I am repeatedly frustrated by the subtle and blatant negative messages we hear from well-meaning but misguided people. It seems to me unnecessary to hand out such pessimism. Why not just recommend preventative measures?

A woman approached me today and asked to speak to me a moment. "My physician has told me," she said, "that I have a high risk for cancer."

In this case, the person did what her physician had failed to recommend. She asked "Do you know of any programs to prevent cancer?"

"Yes, I believe so," I told her. I believe that any programs of treatment having to do with lifestyle, emotion, positive input, and spiritual growth will probably be valuable, not only to help cure but also to help prevent disease of all kinds, including cancer.

What have I been saying? What are the things you can participate in doing to improve your chances of beating cancer? These are the same principles that help prevent cancer.

Here is a "shopping list" of aids to help cure and prevent disease. I am not proposing that you replace medical care with this program, but that you add it to your doctor's regimen. These suggestions will be further developed as you read on.

1. Clarify your purposes for living. We all do better with our lives if we have a "why"!

2. Clarify your personal faith, not in a spiritual being who will exercise total control over you, but one who will love and empower you to work for your own health and well being. Choose the path of peace and love!

3. Seek avenues for spiritual cleansing of bitterness or unforgiveness.

4. Choose joy in life. The best reason for living is that we enjoy it.

5. Develop relaxation skills and use them daily.

6. Remember to breathe! Take at least eight to ten deep breaths three times a day.

7. Use your imagination. Visualize yourself reaching your goal of good health. See your immune system fighting all disease, including cancer.

8. Restructure your negative belief system. Make your fantasies work for you. Make your thought more positive and realistic.

9. Begin a regular, common-sense exercise program.

10. Use good judgment in your diet. Eat plenty of fiber and fruit and vegetables.

Choose life, but remember it is a choice. When or if you become tired and have no more reason, no more "why" to live, you can choose to stop. Such a decision is not to commit literal suicide. It is simply a fact that we can shut down our systems when we are tired of living.

Literature is filled with stories about people who decide to die. There are stories from Eskimo culture about old people who decide life is finished, so they go to a cave or some similar place and die. From prison camps in Korea and Vietnam come stories of people who had lost their sense of purpose and hope. They died from no apparent cause. Certainly there are stories from cancer treatment people and hospitals in general about people who decided there was no purpose, no point to life, no hope. They died too.

When death seems preferable to changing unhealthy life patterns, some people choose to die. A businessman who had bladder cancer is a good example. He went on a stress reduction program. He lightened his schedule, re-laxed, and began an exercise program. The tumor shrunk.

He came into my office one day and said, "I know that if I continue this reduced schedule, I can get well and live a long time, but it's not living to me. I'm going back to the heavier schedule at work. I love the stress."

He resumed his former way of life, and the tumor grew again. He died within three months. Stress reduction works, but it is a choice.

The encouraging thing is that choice is involved. If people can choose to die, they can choose to live. If loss or purpose, loss of hope, and a sense of helplessness leads to death decisions, then a recovery of purpose, renewed hope, and a sense of the power from participating in one's own health can lead to life.

• TWO •

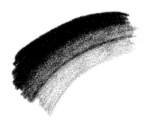

A Profile of a Healthy Person

One of my seminary professors warned me against studying demons. He said, "You become what you study." If he
was correct, we study too many demons. We devote far
too much time and research to sickness and far too little to
health. When do you remember picking up a magazine or
book and reading something like "How I Never Became
Sick" or "The Emotional Profile of a Person Who Has
Never Been Depressed and Never Even Thought of
Suicide"?

When I set out fifteen years ago to do a study on
healthy marriages, I found very little literature on that
topic. Nobody writes an expose about "couples who have
never had marital conflict." No, no! We study sick people
and become what we study. Our books and magazines
describe drug abuse, sexual perversions, suicide, and mental and physical illness. It is no wonder that suicide rates
are up, deviant behavior is rampant, and hospitals are
filled with both physically and mentally ill people.

We should be studying people who are models of physical and mental health. Our students need to see models who are successful and who never used drugs. I want to see some movies about honest, healthy people. The problem is that no one would pay to see them. In fact, we'll continue to see a flood of material on sick society because that is what we buy—a frightening prospect, because we do indeed become what we see modeled.

We have never needed healthy models more. We desperately need to look at the lives of people who are healthy, survivors who are coping with whatever comes along. I recently read about a thirty-nine-year-old man who had established a highly successful business as a stock broker. Then came the October crash of 1987. He was bankrupt. In the midst of business failure, his mental problems escalated. His wife left him. It was too much for him. He pointed a .38 revolver at his temple and pulled the trigger. He had no coping skills, no model for successfully dealing with life's hard blows.

Let's look at people who cope. People who face difficulty and survive, who "keep on keeping on."

Over the last twelve years, I've studied patients who recovered from serious illness, and I've looked at the lives of healthy people who have stood the test of years. I've talked to friends and family members, and from all their observations has come what I call the Healthy Model. The survivors all have some common characteristics. Look at them, copy them, and work your own uniqueness into them.

MAINTAIN BALANCE.

Healthy, coping people are not fanatics, people who, having lost a sense of direction, redouble their efforts. These healthy people have causes. They want to make contributions, but they maintain balance.

Another way of understanding this principle is to see that healthy people view themselves in a lighthearted way. Unhealthy and unhappy people take themselves very, very seriously, and they become upset if everyone, or nearly everyone, doesn't do the same.

My dad is an example of the kind of healthy person I'm talking about. I call him a poor man's philosopher because he never wrote a book nor was he handicapped by too much education. In fact, he attended school for less than eight years. But he never let any of that stop him from expressing sweeping ideas about life.

"I have opinions on prackly everything," he says. "And I'm usually right. At least I think I am, but I guess everyone else thinks he is too."

Dad not only doesn't take himself too seriously, but he helps me not to take myself too seriously too. I asked him for advice in writing a book.

He said, "If you want to write a book, keep it simple, make it entertaining, and don't try to say too much. Most people are like me [one of his basic assumptions], and we want easy entertainment when we read. We don't want to learn a lot. I already know all I want to know. I just read for fun."

Of course, I want this book to be useful. I hope you will find it helpful to you personally. Still, I need to retain enough humility and balance to recognize that a lot of people do read just for fun. That's not all bad. Read on! Enjoying life, in fact, is the best reason for living. Even Jesus taught that He came so that people could have abundant joy.

A few years ago, I talked with Lawrence LeShan. He said that he believes our immune system gives us the raspberries when we ask it to fight for health because we have so much duty and responsibility that we can't be sick. He believes that our immunity really perks up and gets with it when we call it into action because we enjoy life and have too much fun to be sick!

As one person put it, "Life is too important to be

taken seriously." To me this idea means that we shouldn't become upset over personal failure. Don't press too hard. Take time to smell the flowers and trees. Play some, relax more, and dare to go barefoot some of the time. People who wear constant frowns and take themselves very seriously are not usually living healthy lives.

DON'T TAKE YOURSELF TOO SERIOUSLY.

That means that healthy people have a lot of fun. So many of us value laughter as a healing force that Laugh Clinics have sprung up all across this country to help people learn how to laugh. Isn't that sad? We have to be taught how to laugh. If you want to know how natural laughter is, just listen to a bunch of children playing. It is a shame that we forget how to have fun.

My philosophical dad even turns work into fun. "I really have fun at work," he used to say. "I have to spend eight hours a day there, so I am going to have fun, even if I have to aggravate someone else."

Anyone who recognizes that a person's value and worth go beyond the job has reached the top and is free to enjoy life.

HAVING FUN IS HEALTHY.

Laugh a lot, even if you have to do as Norman Cousins did—watch crazy movies. Find funny things and things that are fun to do. If you have a friend you can laugh with, cultivate that friendship. Spend more time with that friend, and stay away from the crepe-hangers. Balance work and play. It is healthy.

I've also noticed that healthy people don't worry, at least not as much. I asked my dad how he handles worry. After his characteristic deep breath and raised eyebrows, he said, "Worry is a word that should be taken out of the dictionary. As long as it is in there, people will think they are supposed to do it. The only reason I can figure for anyone to worry is that he must think it's supposed to be done. If we took the word out of the dictionary, people would stop worrying, and tranquilizers wouldn't sell."

"How about money as a cause of worry?"

"Why, Bill," Dad mocked, "if you have money, you don't need to worry. If you don't have money, you shouldn't waste time worrying about it. You should go out and try to earn some.

"There just aren't many reasons to worry. Dying?" Dad asked the question of himself. "You have known you were going to die since you were this high." He held his hand, palm down, about two feet above the floor. "Since you know it's going to happen, and you can't do anything about it, you might as well go ahead and live while you can.

"Worrying just never made any sense to me," my dad went on. "It never earned a penny, never saved a life, never made anyone well. Right now, I'm worried about being thirsty. Hand me a soda."

That is a practical application of the Serenity Prayer: "God grant me the serenity to accept the things I cannot change, courage to change the things I can, and the wisdom to know the difference."

I obliged Dad with a soda, and he took a drink, smiling as he glanced in my direction. "Now I'm not worried about that anymore!"

WORRY MAKES PEOPLE SICK!

I heard a successful cancer doctor say that the best way to health is to "choose peace, and leave your troubles to God." Worry is useless, but it is worse than that. Worry never solved a problem, and it does make people sick.

Another sign of my dad's good health is his hopefulness in situations that would make most people turn and run. Healthy people believe that there is always a way out, a solution to every problem. When they appear to be trapped, they look for answers, not excuses, and never give in to despair.

Once Dad and I were riding on a two-lane street with

my brother Larry in Chicago. Rain was falling, and traffic was at a standstill. The left lane seemed to open, so Dad suggested that Larry use it.

"We might meet traffic," Larry said.

"Naw," said Dad. "Pull on around this truck. You've got time."

His confidence was so contagious that Larry drove the car into the left lane. Bad decision! Traffic was meeting us head on.

Dad spoke hurriedly with a smile in his voice. "Throw it in reverse."

Larry had obviously decided to go ahead and hope the truck would permit him back in the right lane. "What good will it do to throw it in reverse?" It was more a statement of irritation than a question.

"Well, when they hit you, you can always say you were backing up." My dad grinned as if to say he could always find a way out.

Remember the story about the little boy who found manure under the Christmas tree and started looking for the pony? We'd be healthier and happier if we looked for solutions, for ponies.

People who feel blocked in will give up in despair. People who believe there is a way out will grin and "throw it in reverse." Look for solutions. Look for the bright side. It's good for your health!

THERE IS ALWAYS A WAY OUT!

Healthy people also take responsibility for themselves. As we used to say in Southeast Missouri, "Every tub has to sit on its own bottom."

This is not an easy thing to do. Once at a family reunion, my dad took a terrible ribbing because a few years earlier, he had driven more than halfway from St. Louis to Mississippi and turned around because it was too far to drive at one time.

Later I asked him why he had done that. He said, "I don't think I did."

"Then why didn't you tell them you hadn't done it?"

He thoughtfully replied, "I couldn't do that. Last year I might have told them I did it." If you tell tall tales, you have to pay the consequences.

TAKE RESPONSIBILITY FOR YOURSELF.

I recently was asked what one thing I would say is the single most important advice anyone could give. The most important thing anyone can know, I said, is that she is responsible for herself. This means that each of us has a choice in how to respond to any of life's situations.

If we take responsibility, we will participate in our own health. We'll stop smoking, reduce alcohol intake, cut back on salt, reduce animal fat, maintain healthy weight levels, eat more fruit and vegetables for fiber, vitamins, and minerals, plan stress reduction, exercise regularly, have fun, set goals, establish personal faith, and maintain balance.

People who take responsibility do not wallow in guilt or self-pity. They do not blame others, their race, sex, financial status, or anything else for their own shortcomings.

TAKE WHAT IS AND MAKE
THE MOST OF IT WITHOUT GRIPING.

We follow leaders who say, "I am responsible," and impeach those who say "I am not responsible."

People who accept responsibility for themselves are healthier than the victims who look for ways to suffer.

Of course, this means that healthy people work. They are not lazy. I've never known a healthy person who sat on his "backside."

I asked my dad about work. He said, "Somebody messed this world up before I got here, so I have to work." There's no need to debate that issue. WORK IS HEALTHY. It must be balanced with play, but there is nothing healthy about laziness.

Healthy people also have what I call a practical faith in God. It is a searching, working faith, the kind of faith that works, laughs, and lives responsibly. Faith that doesn't worry, but trusts that somehow there will be a way out. It is a faith that does not claim to speak from God's point of view, but maintains enough humility not to take itself too seriously. (Chapter four, "Healthy Spirituality," talks about this kind of faith in greater detail.)

When problems arise, healthy people ask the right questions. The most important philosophical, theological, psychological question in the world is, "So what?" This question says, "What difference will this make?" When I am concerned about a problem, I ask "Will it matter a hundred years from now?" The right questions help us to keep life in proper perspective. "So what? Who says? Is this worth dying for? What results do I want?"

ASK THE RIGHT QUESTIONS.

"You should do that!"

"Who says?"

"People may not like you."

"So what?"

If you are not getting the answers, it may be that you are asking the wrong questions.

Look at this profile. Let it become a model for you.

• Don't take yourself too seriously.
• Have fun.
• Balance work and play.
• Believe in solutions; look for the way out.
• Work hard.
• Take responsibility for yourself.
• Express your own faith.
• Ask the right questions.

Study healthy people. Read what they read. Model your life after them. Remember that we become like the models that we study.

And now let's turn to healthy beliefs. If your ideas have been causing problems for you, you can change your mind.

• THREE •

You Can Change Your Mind

An extremely perverse woman was in my office recently. I was talking to her about the importance of her thought process as it related to her physical condition. She seemed compelled to disagree with everything I said.

"Your mind and body are connected." I was firm with her.

"No, they aren't." She smirked.

I thought for a minute, trying not to smile. "Well, I guess your mind and body are NOT connected.

She hardly paused to answer, "Well, my brain and body are."

I thought I had her now. "Well, what goes into your brain?"

She almost grinned. "Nothing, when I'm comfortable!"

I think a lot of people believe that nothing goes into their minds or brains, but the fact is that our minds are processing our experience continuously. Everything we see, hear, think, or feel goes into our minds. Whether negative or positive, it all goes into our minds. Everything that goes in will affect us. It is the same as if we were putting data into a computer.

One of my own idiosyncrasies demonstrates the power of that data, years after we absorb it. Until recently, I had difficulty buying shoes. I always felt that I should wait or find a cheaper pair. I would buy shoes at a cut-rate store, on sale, and still feel guilty. Why? Because data (beliefs) had been put into my computer (my mind), and it was kicking out in the form of guilt about buying shoes. Where did these feelings originate?

When I was growing up, my parents, who had little money, repeatedly programmed me. They said, "Take care of your shoes. If you are just going to play, go barefoot, and save your shoes for school or Sunday."

We half-soled shoes, put heels on them, and put taps on the heels and toes. My parents admonished my siblings and me not to "roll our shoes over" or stand on the sides of them, because we couldn't "afford to buy new shoes." Over and over I heard such phrases, so now I don't have to think about them consciously to be influenced by them.

It isn't the money anymore. I could buy an airline ticket to Athens, Greece, and feel no guilt. You can buy a lot of shoes for the cost of an airline ticket to Greece. Yet I bought a ticket without guilt because I have no data concerning that. It never occurred to my parents to tell me not to buy a ticket to Greece.

I have worked to overcome that guilt and have successfully done so by rationally recognizing the process, changing the beliefs, and then acting—in this case, buying shoes. Change the beliefs, then act as if the new beliefs are true.

The point is that what I heard as a child was still influencing me forty years later. Whatever goes into your mind will have an effect on you. You will talk to yourself and affect your attitudes and health by your own self-talk. As Anthony Robbins says in his "Mind Revolution" seminars, "The quality of your life is the quality of your communication to yourself and others." Your communication to yourself is what you say to yourself.

Our minds will register experience, no matter what we do. We cannot control *whether* our minds record mental input, but we can control *what* that input will be. We can deliberately, consciously decide which thoughts we put in our minds.

The question is, what would be helpful? We ought to put healthy, positive thoughts into our minds. Thoughts like those of healthy people will help us to prevent disease and perhaps even help us to overcome disease that is already in our bodies.

We should look at the belief systems of healthy people and deliberately use methods that help us adopt such beliefs as our own. In order to adopt a belief, we must recognize it as a possibility and want to believe it. If we want to make it a part of our own lives, we can do so by following a few simple steps.

1. Identify the negative belief you want to change. State it in order to see it clearly. Then restate the thought in realistic and positive terms.

Suppose, for example, you want to change the belief that you aren't popular. State your negative belief clearly: "I don't have any friends," for example.

Then find a way to express the same idea in a constructive way: "Although I don't have as many friends as I'd like, I have some friends and will gain more friends each month."

It is obvious that anyone would feel better believing the second idea. So start working on it.

2. Now that you have found a positive way of looking at the problem, repeat the new statement.
   Memorize it. Say it aloud. Tell someone else. Say it
   again and again. Repeat the belief to yourself, and
   continue to repeat it until it is firmly entrenched in
   your mind. It helps to write the concept out and
   commit an exact wording to memory.

Every time you think anything contrary to the new
idea, immediately correct even the thought. If someone
else says something stupid to you like, "You don't seem to
have many friends," correct her immediately. Say, "That's
not true. I don't have as many as I'd like, but I do have
some, and I'm steadily gaining new friends all the time."

3. At the same time that you're changing the way you
   talk to yourself about the problem, imagine your
   life the way you would like it to be. Picture yourself enjoying new friends and seeing old ones. In
   your imagination, hear someone saying, "You sure
   seem to be gaining a lot of new friends."

Repeat the new idea until it becomes a possibility in
your mind.

- Repeat it until you believe it probable.
- Repeat it until you believe it.
- Repeat it until it is a conviction.
- Repeat it until you know it is true.

Now it is yours! Keep on reaffirming it.
Practice with other situations:
Negative thought: If she leaves me, I'll never be
happy. I'll always be alone and abandoned.
Positive thought: It would be painful if she leaves me,
but it would not be the end. There are other relationships.
I will make it and I will be happy.
Now use the process. Repeat the positive statement.

Don't accept negative input. Imagine yourself standing strong, and hear yourself saying, "I knew I could be happy on my own."

Repeat it. Repeat it until you know it is true.

Now try another one:.

Negative thought: I am sick. I have cancer (or heart disease, or whatever other illness troubles you). I am going to die.

Positive thought: Of course, I'm sick, but I can get well. Other people have overcome this disease. So can I. I will die, everyone does, but I may not die of cancer. My body will do What Ever It Takes (WEIT) to heal itself.

Repeat it. Repeat it until you know it is true.

One patient told me. "I used to say I'd get well, but wonder whether I would. I just said it because I wanted to believe it. Now I believe it. I know it. I am going to get well." He had lung cancer, with metastases to the brain and bone. Now he has overcome nausea, and his brain is cancer-free. He is getting well.

Through repetition, you can climb the steps, moving from possibility, through probability, belief, and conviction, to knowledge.

KNOWLEDGE
CONVICTION
BELIEF
PROBABILITY
POSSIBILITY

When the belief has become so ingrained that you know it, then it belongs to you.

4. Once you have entrenched a new belief, act as if that belief were true. If we say it and act as if it were true, it becomes part of our own belief system. My buying shoes is an example of acting "as if."

When I was in college, I read about the philosophy of the German thinker, Hans Vaihinger. He based his ideas, which he called Fictional Finalism, on the notion that we all have a belief about life, a fiction that might or might not be true. We then act as if that belief were final and always true.

We may believe, for example, that all tall people are to be feared. This, of course, may be true. If it is true, though, it probably is true only of people over 6'3". The truth of the idea is irrelevant to our behavior. We act as if it were and avoid or hide from all tall people.

Other beliefs, however, are more important to our lives. If I believe that my body is healthy and, within reason, act on that belief, my thoughts can have a positive effect on my health. Here are some beliefs that are life-giving, healing, powerful. They are the beliefs of healthy people, people who have survived serious illness or who avoid disease altogether.

Healthy Belief Number One: "There is healing power in me. My body is working for me. My body is working to fight disease and make me healthy."

If you are a cancer patient, restructure this belief to say, "My body is working to fight cancer. My body will do *What Ever It Takes* to heal itself."

Repeat it, believe it, and act as if it is true.

Healthy Belief Number Two: "My life is worth living. I have as much right to life as anyone. I don't have to prove my worth and value. It is mine because I am a human being. God gives me value, and no one can take it away from me." I suggest that you commit this entire paragraph to memory. It is true.

Your self-image is one of your most important liabilities or assets. If you believe in your own worth and value, there is little you cannot achieve, including better health. No one lives life at a level that is inconsistent with his or her self-concept or self-image.

When I was team psychologist for the St. Louis Cardinals baseball team from 1980-82, I plainly demonstrated the power of our self-image to influence our lives. Player Keith Hernandez has told me many times that he is a .300 hitter. If he's hitting .240, and I ask him what he will hit, he says, "Three hundred." What is his lifetime average? .300! People perform at a level consistent with their self-beliefs.

Phil Bradley, formerly with the Seattle Mariners, for whom I served as team psychologist from 1983-87, hit one home run in his first year in major league baseball. The second year, he hit twenty-six home runs. A huge difference! I asked him what made that difference. He said, "No one ever told me I could hit home runs before this year." Daren Johnson had told him that he could do it. Bradley believed it, and he did it.

What works in baseball also works in our everyday lives. People perform at a level consistent with their self-beliefs. BUT self-beliefs can change, and when they do, their behavior or life changes too. So the way to improve your level of living is to improve your self-concept. Believe in yourself.

After you commit the paragraph on value to memory, start adding some powerful supportive thought. I'll give you a starter list of thoughts and actions to support your growing self-image.

No one can make you think less of yourself unless you permit it. Make up your mind to let no one reduce your view of yourself.

Treat yourself as if you have value. Dress up. Buy yourself a good meal. Treat yourself to a trip. Just treat yourself in general as if you deserve good things.

Read good, encouraging material. Lots of books are designed to help you improve your self-concept. Self-improvement tapes can also help. Listen to them. Read good devotional material too.

Spend time with people who are positive and encouraging. Some people drag you down. They are negative people. They are the takers. They are tiring to be around. You know people like that. Don't hang around them. Someone said that the way to be rich is to find out what poor people read and don't read it! Stay away from draining people as much as possible.

Some other people are exciting and energizing to be around. Hang around with them. Seek them out. Pick their brains. Imitate their lifestyle and beliefs. Spend time with energizers.

Keep on repeating your paragraph on self-worth. Remember, you have as much worth and value as anyone, and no one can take it from you.

Healthy Belief Number Three: "I have purpose. My life has meaning." It is a lot easier to believe this when you act as if it were true. One way to act out this belief is to set some realistic goals for yourself. Make a list of things you want to do. Be free and specific. I think it helps to set goals for one year, two years, five years.

Goals have magnetic power. They attract our energy and move us in directions that enable us to achieve them. Don't be afraid to set goals. They generate health. There are indications in recent health literature that people without purpose are sicker and die faster. Victor Frankl makes this clear in his descriptions of those who died and those who survived the concentration camps of Germany in the 1940s. Similar descriptions came from prisoners of war from Korea and Vietnam. Having a true sense of direction turns on our passion for living. When we restore our passion, our whole system functions better. Believe it and practice.

If you are sick, set a goal for being well. One patient told me recently, "My goal is to be cancer-free in two years." She thought about how she would look and feel then. It was a realistic goal.

If you are well, set a goal to stay well. I plan to play basketball until I'm at least sixty-five years old. I will have to be healthy to do that.

I've talked to people who either think they cannot set goals and find purpose in life, or they are afraid of goals. The fact is, we all set goals for ourselves repeatedly. We just don't call them goals.

When you travel anywhere, you have a destination, a goal. Can you imagine going to an airport and asking the ticket agent for a ticket without a destination?

"A ticket to where?" she'd ask.

"I don't care—just anywhere."

If you were as aimless as that, I'm sure the agent would think you were crazy. I'd agree. You can understand destinations in travel. Whether you make a short trip or a long trip, you have a destination. This can be compared to short-range and long-range goal setting. You can plan a destination.

Goals may also be compared to a planned achievement. You may decide, for example, to go to school to earn a college degree. That's a general goal. Somewhere in the process of education, you must be specific. You cannot get a degree in General.

Imagine someone asking you, "What is your college degree in?"

"I have a Bachelor of Science in General."

"General what?"

"I dunno!"

Are you crazy? No one does that. We all set specific goals if we reach the level of a college degree. The college education is a general goal and the degree a specific goal.

You see, you already know the difference between long-range and short-range goals. You already understand general and specific goals. In fact, you have already set all kinds of goals. I'm suggesting that you write out, or at least think out, some near and some distant destinations for yourself. Make a list of what you want, where you want to be, what kind of person you want to be, what kind of relationships you want. Go over the list and decide which of these goals you will accomplish soon and which require more time.

Now go over the list and turn the general goals into specifics. Describe details as much as you can. Then you can begin to plan for reaching them.

Example: One goal might be to lose weight by one year from now. Is that clear? Of course not. It is, however, a general long-range goal. So make it specific. Suppose I want to lose twenty-six pounds within a year. That means I will need to average one pound every two weeks. Now I can start planning for reaching the goal by working specifically today.

I have been setting goals since I was in junior high school. I knew instinctively that, in order to get somewhere, you have to know where you are going. I set goals in areas of physical conditioning, degrees, and relationships. I wanted to be student body president. It was a goal. I made it! I wanted to set basketball scoring records. I did! I wanted to get a degree from Washington University. I did that too. I wanted to play professional baseball. I never did, but I have worked with major league teams. I decided that was close enough.

We may achieve some things by accident, but usually that is not true. Most achievements we plan on some level. The good news is that you can begin to plan now! Those plans will give purpose to your life and make healthy living more likely.

Healthy Belief Number Four: "I have the right to express myself." Holding feelings inside can be unhealthy. This is especially true when feelings are held in because a person believes he or she has no right to express them. Feelings are not right or wrong. They are just feelings. It is what we do with them that is good or bad. You have a right to express your own feelings.

Healthy Belief Number Five: "I enjoy living." The only reason for living is that we want to live, and we want to live when we have fun. A sense of humor and the ability to find delight in daily living keeps the creative and healthy juices flowing. So in addition to whatever else you do, choose to have fun.

Not everything in life is fun, but most things can be enjoyed. It depends on how you talk to yourself about what is happening to you.

Every day can be a celebration if we make the decision to take whatever we have, whatever we are, and make the most of it. If we do that with the determination not to complain, but to celebrate, we can enjoy life.

Focus as much of your attention as you can on the good and the humorous things in life. Someone once said that God must have had a great sense of humor. He created monkeys, didn't He? He even created some pretty funny people. Most of the time, we can choose to enjoy whatever we have to do.

Healthy Belief Number Six: "I have hope. If anyone can make it, I can." When I asked a cancer patient what was the most helpful thing I had done for her, she said, "You helped restore my hope."

Too often we look at statistics in a damaging way. We say nine of ten die, or seven of ten die. Why not say, "One of ten lives. I can be that one." If we approached statistics that way, we would soon change the statistics.

Remember that there is no such thing as false hope. There is only hope. Real hope! Never be afraid to hope. Believe it! "I have hope."

There is no known illness, no form of cancer from which someone has not recovered. Recovery is always a possibility. It is also true that there has never been a disease that infected everyone who contracted it. In other words, prevention of disease is always possible, and recovery from disease is always possible. There are no hopeless cases. This book is about hope. Hope for cure, hope for prevention, and hope for a better life.

Healthy Belief Number Seven: "I will do *What Ever It Takes.* My body will do *What Ever It Takes* to fight disease." According to Anthony Robbins, this is a belief of successful people in all fields. More than a belief, it is a commitment. I will do *What Ever It Takes* to be creative, to get well, to accomplish whatever it is that I want. *What Ever It Takes*, with the limitation that I will not hurt others.

Healthy Belief Number Eight: "I am in charge of my own life. I am not a victim. I am a participant. I will ask questions. I will put my own thumbprint on this world." This notion clearly suggests personal responsibility. That word may be unpopular, but it is still healthy and unconsciously respected by most people. Consider the alternative. I'm either responsible, or I am a victim.

Healthy Belief Number Nine: "I am a positive person. I do healthy things and think healthy thoughts." The opposite of this belief is clear in the negative thoughts a man expressed to me in a counseling session. "Even when I can have good things, I keep choosing the bad," he said. "I still *always eat the heels* from a loaf of bread, and I don't like the heels. I'm tearing up my car," he added, "because I keep on *driving into the same chuckholes every day.*

A lady told me about her own lonely life on the same day. "I don't answer my phone because *the only time it rings is when it's a wrong number.* Do you blame me for not answering it?"

It looks obvious, but in fact, most of us say and allow negative things into our minds daily. Our prejudice against ourselves is clear.

At a recent seminar, I talked with a group of executives who were at the top in their corporation. I asked them to list their positive attributes and share one or two with the group. Only three of the fifty people present mentioned anything. When I asked for positive things they knew about others, I had to cut off the responses.

They would have responded just as frequently if I had asked them to list their weaknesses.

Please note: It is all right to say good things to and about yourself, no matter what anyone has told you about "bragging." Remember, "Blessed are ye if ye toot your own horn, for verily it shall be well tooted!" It is healthy to say and think positive things about yourself!

The way to establish a belief is through repetition. Write it, say it, repeat it, think it, and act as if it were true. Go over the beliefs of healthy people and make them your own:

- The way to establish a belief is through repetition.
- The way to establish a belief is through repetition.
- The way to establish a belief is through repetition.

• FOUR •

Healthy Spirituality

Are religious people healthier than nonreligious people? I can only speculate, but I suspect that the answer is no. Some religious people may object that such doubts undermine faith. I believe that religion enriches and deepens our lives; it is the expectation that religion be the answer to everything that hurts faith.

I heard a nutritionist recently making just such excessive claims about her vitamin supplement program. It was very effective, she said, against all kinds of ailments, including allergies. The problem was that she was sniffling and wheezing so much. It was hard to understand her, let alone believe her. She had a lot of good things to say, but she hurt her credibility by claiming too much. Religion has a lot to offer, but spokesmen for God sometimes make claims for it that result in a credibility gap.

Let's rephrase the question. Is there a connection between religion and health? The answer to that must be yes. Sometimes the connection is damaging, especially when legalistic religion promotes the negative trinity of extreme guilt, rejection, and fear. But the relationship between religion and health can be positive when it focuses on acceptance and love.

Perhaps the question should be, does healthy spirituality make people healthier? Does it assist in helping people get well? The answer is a resounding YES!

Spirituality may be defined as the belief that there is something more than this material existence. There is meaning beyond this world. There is something greater than the visible world, a creative force, a reality beyond finite life. For some of us, that power is a personal God.

A healthy spirituality includes an ability to believe, to have faith. In describing survivors of cancer, Bernie Siegel says that they have faith in their doctors, faith in themselves, faith in medicine, and faith in God. Faith, the substance of things hoped for and not seen, is an essential ingredient in healthy spirituality, a spirituality that contributes to physical health.

The need for faith in medicine is well documented by myriad studies on the power of placebo. People get sick when they believe a "pill" will make them sick, and they often get better when they believe a "pill" will make them better. In both cases they have been given a sugar pill; the effect is the result of faith, their belief. Certainly faith in your medicine will help you get well.

An active faith in a God of love who wants us to be better physically and wants to free us of pain is certainly more conducive to health than a passive faith in a vindictive God who arbitrarily sends illness on us or punishes us with illness. Positive faith that results in action toward health is a tremendous asset in the healing process and in wellness in general.

Our expectations influence how we weather storms. The widespread publicity about the unpleasant side effects of chemotherapy makes it more difficult for cancer patients to go through treatment without experiencing nausea and other problems. We would be well advised to note that NOT all patients have bad side effects. Belief makes a difference. You may not have any side effects at all.

A healthy spirituality also involves an emphasis on reflective meditation. The quiet times of reflection and personal growth are essential for balance. Healthy spirituality always includes times of solitude. We are discovering that such times permit the physical system to relax and function in a healthier way.

Personal meditation, murmuring to yourself, is essential to maintaining balance. The fast pace must be slowed so that we can examine our ideas. We need a strong philosophy or deep sense of spirituality to cope with life, and that cannot be developed without quiet reflection and decision-making time. This is a tool to use in deciding to punch your "live button." Meditation, relaxation, and prayer contribute to health.

Healthy spirituality is congruent with all of our other attitudes and behavior. That is to say that it fits seamlessly into our lives. It is not phony pietism or pretended strength. It is real, and you can feel the truth of it. You may not agree with another person's convictions, but you respect them if they are real.

When our spirituality fits, it is believable. That fit makes what we say sound real. Believe what you say you believe. Do not pretend something you are not! Do not wear a plastic smile when you are in pain. I do not want to communicate what I am supposed to believe, but what I do believe. The kind of integrity I am talking about encourages healing and health. Living a lie dissipates energy and can make you sick.

Balance, another key concept in producing a healthy life, includes one's approach to spiritual life. Let's consider several kinds of balance that grow out of a healthy spiritual base and see how they relate to good health.

First, there is balance between tolerance of others and

freedom to express one's own faith. Whether you have religious faith or not, you have a right to express your views. For many years, I was reluctant or embarrassed, afraid to express my personal faith. I was tolerant of others, and that was the right thing. I am still tolerant of others. The other side of such acceptance, however, is the expectation of toleration from others.

I have become bolder in my personal expression and more honest in my tolerance in the passing years. There is boldness in healthy spirituality. That is part of the freedom to be one's self.

We mustn't be afraid to say aloud what we are, what we feel, and what we believe in our everyday lives, as I found out when I went fishing on the Gulf of Mexico a few years ago. I was riding in the bow of the boat watching the rolling waves. A queasy feeling came over me. "It's just in my mind," I thought, "and besides, if I do get sick, I'll stay here and never tell my family and that group in the stern."

My pride lasted for about three minutes. Soon I was staggering through the crowd of about thirty people. I was green-faced and had lost all fear of admitting I was sick. I must have shouted, just to remove all doubt, "I'm sick!"

The closer I come to the culmination of life, the less concern I have about appearing to be intellectual or popular. I just want to be real. So I wander through the crowd and say for anyone to hear, "I have faith in God." Healthy spirituality may or may not be a part of an organized religion, but I think it is always characterized by a balance of boldness and tolerance.

On a practical level, it makes sense to be tolerant and flexible. The more flexible and tolerant you are, the more resources you have. Healthy and successful people have alternatives. If you block them, they find an alternate route to their goals, or they find new goals. Whether in religion or work, rigid, one-dimensional people are limited in their responses to life. When such people lose a leg, arm, or breast, they have no options. Their lives are thwarted. Flexible, tolerant people find another area of strength, another direction.

After a terrible motorcycle accident, W. Mitchell proved himself to be just such a creative person. He was burned indescribably. His injuries would have destroyed a rigid person. He would have whined, "Now I can't do what I wanted to do. My life is ruined." Thwarted in the direction he had expected his life to take, W. Mitchell simply changed direction. He became a millionaire manufacturing wood-burning stoves. As if horrible burns were not enough, a plane crash subsequently paralyzed his lower body. Even that disability didn't block him. He is now trying his hand, (what's left of it!) at politics.

Flexible, tolerant people are survivors!

Perhaps flexibility and tolerance are other ways of saying acceptance. Acceptance must be balanced with change. People who survive and live healthy lives accept what comes and are willing to adapt to changing circumstances. They apply the prayer of serenity, a prayer of spiritual balance. They pray for the grace to accept what they cannot change, the courage to change what they can, and the wisdom to know the difference.

Acceptance can make us apathetic victims unless we balance it with a recognition that we are responsible for making life better when we can. A willingness to change implies humility to acknowledge our need to grow and know more. We do not speak from God's point of view. No one does! Acceptance necessitates a willingness to do what we can to make life better for ourselves.

One patient I've seen recently said he had opted to continue chemotherapy after reading Bernie Siegel's book *Love, Medicine and Miracles*. He wants to trust God, but he also wants to make use of what God has provided.

Acceptance does not mean passive fatalism, then. Not

pretending that everything is fine when you are hurting. Acceptance means facing reality. Some would-be spiritual leaders encourage another response, which is a kind of denial. They teach people to ignore illness, pretending that everything is fine with them. They even recommend thanking God for good health without acknowledging sickness. This unrealistic blindness will not stand alongside the Gethsemane faith of Jesus Christ, Who prayed, "If it be possible, let this cup pass from me; nevertheless Your will be done." That is realism coupled with acceptance.

I was asked recently, "Why teach methods of healing and prevention? When it's your time, you're going to die. There is nothing you can do about it." Though that concept is taught by some religious groups and many well-meaning people embrace the concept, it turns people into victims. Worse yet, it is not true.

Sense, unfortunately, is not common, so let's use some uncommon sense. Suppose we experiment to determine the effects of certain behaviors on people's health. Assign ten thousand people to two groups of five thousand each. One group smokes two packs of cigarettes per day, while the other abstains from smoking. If they live similar lifestyles, except for smoking, which group will, on the average, live longer? The nonsmokers, of course! They will live an average of eight to ten years longer. Is it strange that, on an average, "your time will come" earlier if you smoke than if you do not?

You could also use exercise, nutrition or emotional attitudes as variables and find significant differences in the life spans of two groups. You live longer, on the average, if you participate in a moderate exercise program, maintain a balanced diet, or have a positive outlook on life.

Lifestyle clearly has an effect on our general health and our longevity. Healthy spirituality leaves room for personal responsibility and participation in our own health programs. "Trust God, but tie up your camel."

Acceptance does not require that we not try to improve our lives. I worked very hard with a young cancer patient, trying to persuade her to involve herself in her treatment program. I made relaxation tapes for her and encouraged her to visualize health and to exercise. She resisted all my attempts to help, in her honest but misguided faith. She said, "I've prayed, and I believe God will heal me." Maybe God would have healed her, if she had used what she had been given. As it was, she died shortly thereafter.

God gives us a boat and oars, but we have to do the rowing. I accept what is. That is the source of contentment, but I work to make life as good as it can be. The Apostle Paul expressed this idea in Philippians 4, in which he said he had learned to be content, no matter what!

Paul's wisdom brings us to a third characteristic of healthy spiritual living, the presence of peace or contentment. This concept is tricky. Again, finding peace for myself does not mean that I become a victim. It does not mean that I put forth no effort to improve my life. Contentment is a choice. Peace is an inner feeling that results from the ability to make the best of my life situation and then accept the way things are. It is balanced with the stress that results from inactivity. Stress often lets us know we need to change something. Once we make the change, we choose and experience peace.

Contentment doesn't mean I shouldn't leave a bad job, end a bad relationship, or seek to improve my life. It means that I accept responsibility for my decision-making and the decision I make. It means that I have enough sense to recognize what I can do. Having done what I can, I leave my troubles to God and rest.

Making decisions about life is a source of peace. Healthy spirituality encourages us to participate in decision-making. A state of indecision and confusion brings turmoil. If you are struggling with a decision, gather information and decide. You'll be amazed at the peace following that act.

A cancer patient who was experiencing a lot of stress and internal turmoil was struggling with a decision about whether to leave her marriage. One day, she showed up at my office with a smile on her face expressing a real sense of contentment. I knew she had resolved the problem. She said, "I have decided to stay married until the end of June. If things are better then, I'll stay longer. If not, I'm leaving."

Her marriage seems better now, perhaps because of her sense of peace. We cannot predict the outcome of her marriage, but her health is better because of her internal peace.

A friend once told me that peace is turned on at a faucet we cannot reach, but thanksgiving flows from a faucet that is within our grasp. If we turn on thanksgiving, another hand turns on peace. Peace results from decision-making and expressions of gratitude. It grows out of a sense of trust. Peace is healthy! Not only for the individual, but for the world!

Perhaps the deepest and most powerful spiritual characteristic of healthy people is LOVE. Here, we balance our love of self with the love of others, the love of life, God, and the world. Just as we have the freedom to express personal faith, we also are free to express and accept love. Let the lovers of the world confess: We love life! We love ourselves! We love others!

How important is love? It may be the most powerful force in our lives. According to Bernie Siegel, feelings of love and of being loved actually affect our bodies in measurable ways. They lower levels of lactic acid, thereby reducing fatigue. These emotions also raise levels of endorphins, which make people less subject to pain; increase the responsiveness of the white blood cells which naturally protect people against colds and other infections; and reduce the risk of heart attack.

Feeling love even reduces the rate of accidents. Working husbands whose wives kiss them good-bye live longer than those who go without. They also have fewer accidents. It isn't the kiss itself that matters, but the love the kiss expresses.

Love of others begins with an awareness that you are loved. Some people feel unworthy. They think they have to suffer cancer or some other problem in order to "deserve" love. They believe they have to hide their scars in order to be loved. NOT TRUE!

Jesus said we are to love our neighbors as we love ourselves. How do you love yourself? A good way is to think of three or four things to do for someone you love and then do something similar for yourself. You might write your friend a note, buy her a gift, and take her out to dinner or to a show.

It might sound silly, but I'm serious in suggesting you do those things for yourself. Write yourself a note of encouragement, buy yourself a gift, take yourself to dinner. Invite a friend to go with you if you like. Be creative and extravagant in expressing love to yourself. Then love others as you love yourself.

Permit yourself to fall in love with life, with all of nature. Let walking in the park be a spiritual experience. Stop worrying about what anyone else would think, and be yourself. Let yourself love all creation freely. John Milton, the poet, wondered whether earth might be "but the shadow of Heaven." What if we are only symbols of ourselves here on earth, and our real being is somewhere else, perhaps in the heart of God?

It is the spiritual and healing experience of love that empowers us to let go of those things that block health and wholeness and cling to the things that anchor us to what is best in life.

When you begin to accept and experience love, especially and particularly unconditional love, you begin to learn some exciting things about life. Note that unconditional love is love that does not have to be earned. It loves, regardless of defects, and everyone has a right to it. It is the kind of love I experienced from my Grandmother Little. She loved me no matter what. She didn't approve of everything I did, but I never doubted her love.

I wish everyone could have that kind of love from someone. We'd all be healthier if that were true. That experience begins with our feeling that we deserve and can have that kind of love. Christians believe that God loves us all, even when we are unlovely. If all Christians acted on that belief, there would be more Christians.

Once you grasp this fact and begin to love yourself, love others, love life, and accept love for yourself, you discover a restoration and strengthening of hope. I never will forget the cancer patient who turned his treatment around and survived the odds. I loved him, and he loved me. I asked, "What was the most important and powerful thing you learned here?"

"That I had hope!" he said. "You helped me restore my hope."

Hope is a result of believing you have a chance to live and succeed. It is a result of goals and directions. It is the belief that the human being has been given a miraculous gift, a body that will do whatever it takes to recover, if we free it to work in spiritual strength. Realistic hope recognizes the work to be done and accepts all the sensible help it can get. It is a healing force, and it grows in the hot house of love.

Love also reduces fear, a debilitating, costly emotion. Fear of rejection keeps us from reaching out to others. Fear of failure keeps us from trying new things. Fear of pain prevents our crossing the threshold to peace. Fear of death obstructs our living.

Love casts out fear. The Bible teaches that perfect love casts out all fear. When I am afraid, I remember arms of love around me; I remember the tender looks of love. I remember the words of encouragement and love, and I am not afraid.

Sometimes I slip back in my mind to early childhood experiences to feel loved. One night, after I had been talking to some people about heart attacks, I felt a pain in my chest. Maybe this was it, I thought. I was alone. Should I write a final note? Should I try to call for help? Should I wait? "Oh, God," I thought, "what if I'm dying?"

I was on the edge of panic when I remembered my childhood, when I prayed with my grandmother, "Now I lay me down to sleep. I pray the Lord my soul to keep. If I should die before I wake, I pray the Lord my soul to take. God bless my family. Amen."

As I returned in my imagination to the care of my grandmother, I soon drifted off to sleep on memories of love that casts out fear.

Love also equalizes guilt, and who doesn't feel some guilt? We all have a fair claim to a bit of it. It is, however, a useless emotion. It seems to have only two values. First, we often resist temptation because we know what guilt a wrongful act will cause. That is a constructive use for guilt, to prevent our doing what we believe is wrong, and to motivate our doing what is right. But this is not the most common use of guilt.

We also use guilt to salve our consciences when we have misbehaved. "Well, yes," we tell ourselves, "I lied, but I feel guilty. If I were not such a good person, I wouldn't feel guilty."

Excuses are useless, of course, but love tells us that we can be forgiven for anything if we are truly sorry and honestly mean to do better. We should accept others' forgiveness as a gift. We should extend it with open hands to those who have hurt us in some way. Yet we withhold forgiveness and embrace resentment instead.

Resentment is like a burr in your pocket. It pricks you every time you sit down on it, and by the time you put it under someone you "have it in for," its sharpness has been dulled on your own backside. It always hurts you more than it hurts anyone else.

If you are holding resentment, release it. Telephone the person you resent or write to him. You don't have to become "bosom buddies." Just let go of resenting him. If the person is deceased, write him a letter anyway. Express yourself.

Forgive him for real or imagined hurts and symbolically burn the letter, letting the smoke soar into the heavens to cleanse your own soul.

Love makes us thankful, too. I am thankful for every day of life. I love to thank people for their encouragement and help, and in that thanksgiving, a wonderful thing happens. Try it. Next time you feel tense and worried, sit down. Take a deep breath. Then slowly start listing all the things for which you feel thankful. You will experience a sense of peace and joy that goes beyond your understanding.

Now we've made the circle. We're back to peace and joy, those spiritual twins that energize life and health. They cure and prevent disease.

EXPRESS FAITH. DARE TO LOVE. LET GO OF FEAR, GUILT, AND DESPAIR. DARE TO HOPE. EXPRESS GRATITUDE.

Joy and peace flow from invisible sources we cannot control. But we can reach love, forgiveness, and gratitude. Turn those emotions on, and the unseen hands of others, or God, will turn on peace and joy as well.

Joy is vital to healthy living. Walter Russell called joy one of the five keys to success and the crowning key. When he speaks of joy, he doesn't mean the superficial appearance of the "hail fellow, well met with a smile," but deep satisfaction and happiness that comes from a sense of self-worth and self-respect.

True spirituality is never a matter of outward ritual or

legalistic rule following. It is certainly not limited to organization or institutional religion, though it is frequently found there. True spirituality is a matter of the heart. It is healthy and healing. I know of no more valuable attitude for prevention of disease and healing of disease than this kind of spirituality.

In my study of cancer patients, the longtime survivors said remarkable things to me about the power of spiritual strength.

"I used to feel ugly because of marks on my face," said one woman. "Now I laugh about them. When I start to get depressed, I pray and read the Bible. The health program you described [now outlined in chapter two of this book] helped me to realize that cancer does not equal death. I am going to get a job, to keep occupied instead of sitting."

This woman had learned to use her sense of humor, her joy of living. She had become an active participant in her own health care. She was trusting God, but doing all she could herself as well. That is true spirituality.

• FIVE •

Becoming What You Behold

I once read a story about a young prince who was deformed. Because of a crooked back, he stood in an awkward posture. The king commissioned a sculptor to make a statue of the prince. In his imagination, the sculptor delivered the crippled prince from his deformity. He gave the statue regal bearing and a handsome, healthy appearance.

Every day for months, the prince sat in the garden, gazing at the image of what he might have been. He dreamed of looking like that. So gradually that he hardly noticed, he stood more and more erect, until one day, he looked into a mirror, and there was looking back at him the image of a man standing straight and tall. As he had gazed at the statue, he had become like it.

We become visions of ourselves. What we see is not only what we get, but also what we become. The dreams, images, or visualizations that we hold consistently in our mind's eye influence drastically what all of us get in life.

Like the prince, we need healthy models. What visions fill your imagination? Are they visions of heart attacks, cancer, accidents, losing, failing, being fired, being cheated on or lied to? How many nights have you finally drifted off to sleep after building horror stories about the things that might happen the next day?

Right now, determine to stop that.

One of my clients persistently sees negative visions on the screen of her mind. She was unsuccessful in turning them off, so she had to learn to ignore the picture or change the channel. She consciously substituted positive thought. When negative images show up in your mind, you can change channels too.

We would all be healthier if we spent time drawing mental pictures of ourselves being healthy and successful, winning and having fun, being loved and encouraged.

The power of visual images has been well documented. Sick people who have consciously envisioned new images of themselves have been able to improve their health. The benefits of visualizing techniques have also been dramatically clear in the performance of professional athletes.

One major league pitcher with whom I worked was at a dead end in his career. He could not control his pitches. He started using relaxation and visualization. Three times a day, he relaxed and listened to an audio tape I made for him. The tape talked him through a visual exercise in which he saw himself from the time he got a signal for a specific pitch from the catcher, through his windup and delivery. He saw himself in perfect form and balance and then saw the ball arriving in the strike zone, right where he wanted it.

In several newspaper stories, he credited that process with saving his career and making him an All-Star pitcher. "Without this help," he said, "I'd be hanging drywall instead of pitching for a salary of six figures a year."

Other professional baseball players, not only pitchers, but also catchers and hitters, echo this story. The improvement in their performance is easy to measure and easy for observers to see. The same techniques that these athletes found to be so helpful are easily adapted to use by people who are suffering from cancer and other diseases.

To visualize is to imagine that you can see images, even if at first you cannot. Some people close their eyes and see images. Others see nothing, but they can create word pictures. These are different ways of visualizing.

I ask my clients to use imagination and practice visualizing for two reasons. First, when you form a clear visual image of anything, you increase the likelihood of its becoming a reality. An image becomes a vision or a pictorial goal and acts like a magnet, moving our life energy toward it. If you imagine yourself healthy and picture in your mind what that would be like—if you see yourself enjoying a social outing, playing a game, dancing, running, exercising—you are much more likely to achieve health.

Many cancer patients use this process to help restore health to their bodies. They picture their white blood cells, the workers in the immune system, fighting cancer. Each person uses her own unique pictures. Some see their white cells as piranha fish attacking and destroying the cancer cells in their bodies. Others see the immune system functioning like PacMan in a video game. Others see armies of medical people in their blood, working for healing. Some picture God sending power for recovery. Whatever the symbolism, the people who practice seeing these images three or more times every day seem to do better consistently in fighting cancer than those patients who do not participate in their healing programs through imagination.

The second reason I recommend using your imagination is that, if you cannot imagine a thing, you cannot believe it, and without being able to believe it, you have no hope. Hope energizes us.

In a sense, then, seeing is believing. And our beliefs shape our emotions, reactions, and behaviors. To practice visualizing is to practice seeing is to practice believing— and belief shapes our lives.

The process is a simple and powerful one. Decide what you want. Picture it and practice seeing it at least three times a day.

THE PROCESS WORKS, BUT YOU MUST WORK IT.

Many start, few finish. A lot of people make short-term gains with the use of visualization, then quit. They become bored or tired, and they lose motivation. If you want something—a house, a wife, a job, good health— enough to work at it, there is no reason to become tired or bored. There is nothing boring about getting what you want! We daydream continually anyway; we might as well use our imaginations in constructive ways.

Many people enjoy the process. "I like visualization," one cancer patient told me. "I used visualization during radiation, and at other times almost every day. I imagined my vocal cords "de-swelling," because I am more concerned about my voice than about cancer returning. I have learned that I tend to let outside factors influence my emotions too much. I'm working on that problem now. And I imagine my body fighting all infections."

The process worked remarkably well for this singer. "My hair is growing back, and my singing voice is maybe sixty per cent of the way back to normal. I am much stronger mentally now than before the program. I believe I can handle most anything."

She thought about her father, who had died two years earlier. "I wish he could have known about these methods," she said. "I really feel strengthened by the program. I am a Muhammed Ali in my fight against cancer. I am not afraid."

Her desire, not only to stay alive, but to LIVE in the fullest sense of the word, is clear in the singer's conversation. Her fighting spirit and her desire to live are evidence of healthy spirituality. They are powerful resources in recovery from disease.

No one seems to understand how, but the evidence indicates that this process of visualizing in many cases empowers the system to fight cancer more effectively. The fact that we don't understand the "how" is irrelevant. When Sir Alexander Fleming found that a little mold spore had landed in his experiment and killed off bacteria in a circle around the spore, he didn't understand the mechanism. He knew, though, that penicillin might be a powerful agent in fighting disease.

I've never understood how TV works, but I've watched it for more than thirty years. Don't wait until you understand imagery or visualization to use it.

• SIX •

Celebrate Life

Human beings celebrate all sorts of occasions. At the birth of a baby, we celebrate by taking pictures, sending and receiving cards, and happily telling anyone who will listen about "the" baby. We celebrate graduation, anniversaries, and all kinds of accomplishments. We celebrate victories and sales. We celebrate holidays. We celebrate autumn— and friends and our connection to a school—with homecoming games and bonfires.

Look at all the ways we celebrate. We eat, dance, yell, laugh, sing, and tell. When celebrations are not used as occasions to abuse chemicals or corrupt our bodies, they are fun and healthy.

It surprises me that so few people think of just celebrating life. We don't have to wait for a special occasion. Celebration is so healthy that we need to plan or schedule regular celebration in our lives.

If you are a parent, celebrate with your children. For no reason other than your love for them, create a special moment for them. One person I know went to school and picked up her son at midday. She took him to a local planetarium, the place he chose for an outing. It was a celebration neither the mother nor the child will ever forget.

Celebrating also means doing nice things for yourself. Take yourself to a movie, buy yourself a gift, or just go someplace you've wanted to visit. Build into your regular routine a special time for yourself at least once a week.

To help others celebrate, do specials things for them. Don't wait for a reason. Make a reason!

Such gestures manifest our love and appreciation for others in our lives. We can also celebrate in more fundamental ways. Probably the number one need for celebrating life is simply to be conscious. It is really ironic that many professionals spend so much time trying to learn how to put people into a hypnotic trance when most of us live in a trance all the time, unaware of what people say to us, unaware of what we just read, unaware of what is happening in the world around us.

The real challenge facing us is not to induce trances, but how in the world to get ourselves out of them. Pay attention now. When I count to three, you will awaken. One...two...three. I hope that worked, because, in order to celebrate life, you must be conscious.

Some people live in a trance so deep that others cannot reach them. Recently a woman was complaining in my office that a man didn't listen to her. She said, "He won't listen to me because I am a woman and because he doesn't consider me important enough."

Then she mused, as if thinking aloud, "That shouldn't upset me, though, since HE DOESN'T EVEN LISTEN TO HIMSELF."

That's really something, isn't it? Some people are so unconscious that they not only do not listen to others, they don't even listen to themselves. WAKE UP! You really miss a lot by walking around like a zombie, sitting in front of a television set until you turn into a "couch potato," or drugging yourself into oblivion. You owe it to yourself to be conscious.

Often as I begin a lecture, I say to the audience, "Now I commit myself to being fully present for this presentation. I want to experience these moments as fully as I possibly can."

I owe it to myself and others to be present. I hate missing now, because it is all I will have to remember tomorrow.

I AM CONSCIOUS!

I AM PRESENT!

I CELEBRATE THIS PRESENT MOMENT!

Once you are conscious and present in the "now," you celebrate by taking what is, and making the most of it without complaining. What a waste when we spend our energies bemoaning what we don't have and where we are not. You can never celebrate life if you constantly compare your lot with that of other people and complain about your life...your spouse...your job...your home...your car....

Begin the celebration. Turn today into a party by taking what you have and determining to make it the best you possibly can. Do that without complaining, and you will experience an immediate sense of joy. Paul the Apostle said he had learned the secret of happiness in the truth that he could be happy or content no matter what his outward circumstances. Make the most of your situation. It is all that you have.

Determine to have fun in the here and now. Love yourself to find ways to give yourself pleasure. That is not a selfish thing to do. You cannot care as much as you should unless you are kind to yourself. You do not have energy to give to others unless you feel good about you. Ethical systems are built on the admonition to love others as you LOVE YOURSELF.

One necessary part of having fun and celebrating life

is the decision to deliberately spend time with people who are fun. Avoid people who drag you down. Come back to them only after you have gained strength through association with "up" people.

Remember that loving yourself involves things like taking time for a hot bath, sending yourself a nice or funny card, buying yourself a gift, taking time for reading a good book, listening to your favorite music, going for a walk or a drive, shopping, playing a game, calling a friend. . .doing anything that gives you pleasure. I know that you don't have time to do nice things for yourself. TAKE TIME! That's what loving yourself and others is all about.

When you celebrate, share the joy. Never make the mistake of not sharing your life with the other people who matter in your world. Treat people as ends and not means to an end.

I heard recently the story of a porter at an airport who was suffering verbal abuse from a businessman.

When the man had vented his spleen, a bystander approached the porter and said, "You certainly are to be commended for your patience with that man."

The porter smiled. "It was nothing," he said. "I just try to be a gentleman." He winked. "And anyway, he is going to Florida, and his bags are going to Michigan."

If we treat people as a means to an end, as objects, we lose sight of their value. That attitude will come back to us. What goes around comes around! You cannot really celebrate life unless you value the people around you and share life with them. Who ever heard of a party with no one there?

We celebrate life, too, through gratitude. Be thankful. Express your thanks to others and to yourself. You can even celebrate the healthy functioning of your body, instead of taking it for granted.

A lady came to see me a few weeks ago complaining

of severe pain in her lower back. In addition to the pain, she was afraid, not only of possible surgery, but even of the diagnostic tests.

We started using relaxation and visualization to help her body to fight the condition. She made gradual progress, with some reduction in pain.

One day she came in and reported that she was better. She had been able to work her full shift with minimal pain, but felt very tired when she got home.

"Be sure and celebrate your body's work," I said.

"What do you mean?" she asked.

"When you arrive home after a good day with minimal pain, say to your body, 'Thank you for a good job today. You deserve a rest so I'm going to give you some time to recuperate. Thank You!'"

She did it every day, and, in one week, she reported dramatic improvement—the best week she'd had in a year. Coincidental? I don't think so.

We would be wise to carry on encouraging conversations with our bodies. The Russians have a proverb: "The mind and body converse, and sometimes the conversation is deadly." The conversation can be healthy if we make it a celebration.

There are special ways that individuals find for personal celebration. When I feel peace and serenity, I like to celebrate with poetry. One poem, "Fireflies," celebrates hope:

> I'd like to grasp
>   that flickering light
> And hold it in my clenched
>   fist tight.
> Then in the hour of deepest
>   darkness for me,
> I'd open my hand and
>   be able to see.

Poetry gives me the opportunity to celebrate my world, my family, and myself. Other people find other ways of expressing their joy.

• SEVEN •

How Do You Know the Facts

How do you know what to believe about your health? What causes cancer? What treatment is best? How can we prevent disease? Most people don't read research or even care about it. We trust others to read and interpret for us. Even though NO ONE CARES AS MUCH ABOUT OUR HEALTH AS WE DO.

Let's take the gloves off and talk about this issue. What difference does it make to you whether you participate in your medical care? Let's look at some examples.

Suppose you are a woman who has just been diagnosed with a malignant lump in your breast. Your physician has told you that the best thing is to schedule immediate surgery...have a modified radical mastectomy... remove the breast. Do you have options?

If this happens to you, I suggest that you get at least one or two more opinions. Your surgeon probably does not expect that reaction. He may not expect you to ask questions at all; some people still expect women to be submissive to men, especially to doctors. You might even have a doctor who refuses to answer questions. He might say things like, "I'm the doctor. I know what's best for you." If that happens, go to another doctor. You have the right to ask questions and to seek second opinions.

Specifically, ask about lumpectomy. For the last four or five years, the research reported in the *Journal of the American Medical Association* and the *New England Journal of Medicine* has shown that lumpectomies for cancers up to four centimeters (about the size of a quarter), coupled with radiation, are just as effective as mastectomies.

Don't accept anybody's views, including mine, on authority. Listen to several voices. One person worth listening to, the voice of experience, Judy Hunt, is a woman I know who spoke up to doctors in her own behalf. Listen to her story as Judy herself tells it in a letter:

"The most important responsibility any person has is her own personal health. My own recent experience confirmed for me the ultimate significance of that responsibility.

"Sensing that there was something medically wrong, I questioned my gynecologist during an annual checkup. He suggested that I was unduly concerned, especially since my age and background did not provide any of the traditional warning signs of cancer. Humoring me, nevertheless, he dutifully requested a mammogram and telephoned a week later to tell me, 'All clear. No problems. Come back next year.'

"I respected his professional opinion, but I knew there was a slight increase in the size of my left breast and I also knew that change is one of the signs of cancer. I decided to consult a medical oncologist who had treated my close friend for two years—a highly respected cancer specialist with long experience. After seeing my recent mammogram and examining me, he chided me for seeking attention. 'There's no cause for alarm,' he said. 'Go home, and don't worry. Take care of your friend.' He cautioned that women my age should have a mammogram every year or two and told me to come back then.

"Not yet satisfied, I returned to my gynecologist, repeated my concerns, and asked whether he could do some additional test. His second examination was coincidentally on the tenth day after the beginning of a menstrual period, the day which I later learned is most reliable for a breast exam. This time, he felt something he called a 'possible lump.' He suggested that we wait for six months to see whether there might be any change.

"Realizing that, if the mass were malignant, time was of the essence, I pressed for more information and immediate further tests. The gynecologist reluctantly described a needle aspiration test that might allow him to distinguish between a fluid-filled cyst and a solid tumor. He remained firm in his opinion that there was no immediate need for that test, but if the lump were still there in a few months, he would do the aspiration then. Not willing to tolerate the wait, I directed him to aspirate the mass now. He complied, just to appease me and get me out of his office. Preparing to do the test, he described the green fluid I would soon see.

"As the procedure progressed, I observed the changing expression on my doctor's face. He didn't have to tell me that there was no fluid. We now began to discuss the difference between benign and malignant tumors. I listened politely to his explanation of the reasons this one was probably benign. He recommended the non-alarmist approach of observing the mass for a few months. I decided that I did not want any tumor, malignant or benign, in my body. I wanted it removed immediately. This day was a Friday; a surgeon recommended by my gynecologist scheduled the biopsy for the following Monday.

"My worst fears were realized when, following the biopsy, the surgeon said the word 'malignant.' Painful as that knowledge was, enlightenment enabled me to act. I listened while the surgeon described the tumor in technical terms and expressed his professional opinion that the only appropriate treatment in my situation was a mastectomy within the week. When I disagreed, he told me to go home and think about the matter, and then come back to his office the following afternoon.

"When I returned, I asked about alternatives to total mastectomy. He advised me that, because of the tumor's size, I was not a candidate for lumpectomy, and reiterated that the best approach was immediate mastectomy. I asked about blood tests and tissue tests to indicate the rate of the tumor's growth. The surgeon told me that he could order these tests only as pre-operative procedures, and only if I agreed to accept the surgery within three days. I signed the consent form and went to the lab for the tests. The following day, I called the lab for the results, spoke to the pathologist about the doubling time of my tumor, and then cancelled the surgery. Now I had the information with which to pursue a second opinion.

"Knowing that a decision this important must be an educated one, and having been acquainted with the Cancer Information Center at Barnard Cancer Center in Barnes Hospital, I immediately drove to Barnes, picked up all the materials relating to breast cancer, and went home to read. I found literature suggesting that tumors under two centimeters could be treated successfully with a lumpectomy followed by radiation, with the same prognosis as that following a total mastectomy. A telephone conversation with a top radiology oncologist confirmed my view that I was a good candidate for a lumpectomy. Three weeks after the date my first surgeon cited as the latest possible time any productive surgery could be performed on me, I underwent a second operation to remove the tissue around the tumor and underarm lymph nodes. At the same time, the surgeon implanted material which was temporarily radioactive, to kill any stray cancer cells. I have a ninety-five percent likelihood of no recurrence. And I still have my own two breasts, with only one small scar to show that the left one was once cancerous.

"A few weeks later, I went with my friend to the office of the medical oncologist who had told me, 'Go home, don't worry, and come back in a year or two.' After hearing my story, he said, 'I'm really glad you handled it the way you did.'

"I don't want to discredit any physician," Judy writes, "but I wish to encourage the reader to accept the ultimate responsibility for her own personal health. You are the person most qualified to make decisions relating to your body. To make such decisions, you must learn all the options available to you."

If Judy had listened to her first two doctors, she might now be dealing with tumors that had spread beyond the breast to the rest of her body. If she had let the surgeon intimidate her, she would have lost a breast needlessly.

Not everybody, of course, is able or willing to go to such lengths as Judy did. But her story illustrates several of the major points in this book. No one is more concerned about your health than you are. Second, you will be wise to seek more than one opinion when you are facing a major medical problem. And, finally, you can be an active participant in your medical treatment. It is your body! Ask questions and get involved in the decision-making process. Judy did, and she is glad!

I asked a physician friend why some surgeons continue to recommend and perform mastectomies routinely when lumpectomies would be as good or better for the patient.

"Because some doctors have twenty-five years of experience," he said, "and some have one year's experience twenty-five times. The latter are the problems."

My own suspicion is that the practice would change drastically if more surgeons were female.

George Crile, M.D., founder of the Cleveland Clinic and author of several books on surgery, told me in 1980 that "there is virtually no reason now for any woman to lose her breast." He further said that, when Halsted invented the mastectomy in the late nineteenth century, there were no radiation treatments available. Crile believed that, after ninety years, the practice should be changed. (Perhaps one year's experience can be repeated ninety times!) What should you do? Ask questions, and, if possible, read the results of research.

Let's look at another example. Suppose your doctor has diagnosed a blockage in your arteries and says that you need a triple bypass operation. What can you do?

Get a second opinion? Probably, unless you are already experiencing chest pain and are in immediate danger. I might be tempted to call someone anyway. Ask questions? Damn betcha! Ask about the recommended surgeon's success rate with that operation. Are there other doctors with a better success rate? How many heart operations does the hospital do in a year? Mortality is much lower in hospitals where heart surgery is routine. Ask your general practitioner or an internist or anyone who has medical knowledge.

If you can, read about alternatives. Now there are some. Less radical procedures might be better for you. Ask doctors working in various specialties. You know what they say; if you give a person a hammer, he'll treat every problem like a nail. A surgeon usually recommends surgery.

Many people, even many experts, are misinformed. How do you know what to believe? For that matter, how do you know that this book is reliable? I did a seven-year study at a research hospital, involving fifty cancer patients with various types and sites of cancer: "Emotions, Stress,

Quality of Life, and the Response of Cancer Patients in Treatment." You can look up that study in a university library; read it, and judge for yourself.

We used random numbers to assign patients to two groups. It is important that patients were randomly selected, to avoid bias and ensure that we wouldn't pick healthier or more assertive patients for either group.

If you ever read a scientific paper, remember that the people in the "control group" are not given whatever treatment is being studied. The second group, the "experimental group," receive the treatment, drug, procedure, or whatever else the researchers are testing. The scientists compare the responses of the control group and the experimental group.

In our research, we tested the value of relaxation, visualization, exercise, and positive thought-formation. The experimental patients continued with their regular treatment plus this program.

We used tests to determine changes or differences in the two groups. Although there were very few, the differences we found really mattered. The experimental group lived longer, and they were more likely to remain free of cancer. At the end of seven years, 84 percent of the experimental group were still alive, compared to 46 percent of the control group. The experimental group's chances of survival for seven years were 59 percent better than the chances of the control group.

It is important to understand that the results are NOT conclusive. More research needs to be done. The direction of the research, however, has led me to believe that the principles we tested really helped our patients. I further concluded that, if these practices help cancer patients, THEY CAN HELP EVERYONE. And if these practices help people to overcome disease, they can help PREVENT disease.

I hope this book helps cancer patients, but I hope also

that the principles will be applied across the board to help people with other health problems.

Still, I know that people find it hard to stick with a discipline, even when they know it's good for them. Could it be true, as some people think, that we would rather be victims than take responsibility for our health? Do we prefer surgery to responsibility? We certainly suffer from a lot of diseases of choice, diseases resulting from our decisions to smoke, overeat, eat unhealthy food, avoid exercise, ignore stress, and drink too much alcohol. Our choices can bring many serious ailments upon us.

I recently heard Dr. Kenneth Cooper, the physician who founded the Aerobics Center in Dallas, Texas, talk about the way we live. "Age slowly or age rapidly," he said. "It's up to you. You can choose a lifestyle that will enhance your health."

Oh, I know. We all are going to die, and we are going to die soon. That's possible, but it is also possible that a lot more of us could live longer and die healthy!

• EIGHT •

The Last Word

There are some things I believe strongly. As far as my experience goes, I know them.

I am certain that people will be healthier if they practice regular relaxation. If that is combined with regular deep breathing and periods of meditation on positive things, all the better. Relaxation does not hurt people. It helps. You will have a better chance of avoiding disease if you practice relaxation. Even if you are not sick, practice relaxation at least twice a day. (Specific instructions are on pages 78-80.)

Two and a half years into his "three months of life," I asked Dave what had helped him most in this adjunct treatment program.

"I'm more relaxed about life," he said. "I practice relaxation with an audio tape three times a day . . . I'm able to flow with life. That is one very important benefit to me."

I am certain that picturing health through visualization and word pictures helps people get well and stay healthier. I sometimes imagine myself running or shooting a basketball when I'm sixty-five years old. I suspect that when I'm sixty-five, I'll imagine doing those things at seventy or seventy-five. That image is healthy, because, in order to make it come true, I will have to be healthy.

I imagine myself trim, a lean, mean machine. That picture implies that my diet be good and my exercise sufficient. Picture health in whatever way works for you. Use your imagination—wake it up and dust it off.

Our dreams have a way of coming true. In the words of the poet, "I dreamed a dream and set it asail/ I dreamed a dream, and dreams don't fail." I am an optimist, so even if a dream failed temporarily, I'd dream it again. I imagine. I visualize. I dream of health and wholeness.

I am certain that exercise, at least a moderate aerobic exercise program, helps people. Since the exercise craze of the late sixties, we've seen a steady decline in the incidence of strokes and heart attacks. The average age of heart attack victims is on the rise, according to Dr. Kenneth Cooper. Our bodies function better when we exercise them than when we let them atrophy in front of the TV. We can eat and laze our way into an early grave.

I am certain that participating in our own health care is better for us than assuming the role of victim. The patients with whom I work consistently affirm the importance of participation. They unanimously echo the words of a breast cancer patient.

"In addition to relaxation and goal setting," she says, "one of the most important things I've learned in the adjunct treatment program is that I am involved in my own health care. It gives me a sense of strength and at least some measure of control."

We have been so afraid of inducing guilt by telling people that they participate in their diseases, and thus in their health, that we kill them with kindness. We hurt people if we tell diabetics that they have no responsibility for their diet. We damage patients who have oat cell carcinoma of the lungs when we pretend that smoking was not really their fault. Holding in anger and anxiety and dealing inappropriately with such emotions is unhealthy. Drinking alcohol injures the alcoholic.

No, we do not directly choose to have cancer, high blood pressure, strokes, ulcers, heart attacks, and other illnesses. But we CERTAINLY choose the LIFESTYLES that lead to them. The good news is that, since we are involved in sickness, we can be involved in getting well and staying well. It is healthy to be an active participant.

I am certain that a clear and specific philosophy and healthy religious faith have beneficial effects on our health.

Dave continued answering the question about benefits from our adjunct treatment program. "I now have a more clear conviction about God," he said. "I believed in God before I began this program, but it was a kind of general faith. Now I have a personal relationship with my God. That has helped me."

Never be ashamed of your spiritual life. It gives depth to your existence and helps you stay well.

I am certain that a sense of purpose is healthy. Life means going somewhere. The direction is up to you. Set goals. There is magnetic and energizing power in purpose, in goals.

If I get on a plane, I want to know where it is going. Well, on this trip through life, I want to know where I'm going, so I set goals. Goals give me a direction and a purpose. I instruct my clients to set goals and, when they begin to achieve them, to re-set them. Always keep something in front of you that is worth living for, and maybe you WILL live!

I am certain that having fun is healthy. Laughing is relaxing. Laughing is energizing. Laughing is a pain-killer. You'll live longer and be healthier if you have fun. Enjoy life! Read a joke book, see a funny movie, or look at yourself in the mirror. Find a way to have fun.

I listened recently to a child's view of some of our

history. One child wrote about the Reformation: "Martin Luther was nailed to the door of the church at Wittenburg. That later led to his death, and he remained dead to this day." I laughed at that. Remember that life is too important to take seriously. Laugh a little. It's healthy.

I am certain that positive attitudes and thoughts are healthy too. Norman Vincent Peale is right. There is power in positive thinking.

I am not an unrealistic Pollyanna skipping through life. Pain is real to me, sickness is real, sorrow is real. But so is comfort, so is wellness, so is joy. Since I live in my own thought, I'll make my home in the land of positives. I choose to think positively, and I believe that is healthy. Accentuate the positives!

I am certain that a high-fiber, low-fat, regulated diet is healthy. We are what we think and what we eat. Some people are big negative cheeseburgers. I want to be a positive apple. Maybe a mixture of fruit. Proper diet reduces cholesterol, shrinks ulcers, and eliminates swelling hemorrhoids. Proper diets that include fruit, vegetables, fish, and poultry are healthy. If you eat right, you live longer and healthier.

I am certain that love and encouragement are healthy. Fall in love with life, with your family, with God, with the world. When you are in love, you feel better. I don't mean only romantic love. I mean love that cares about life and people.

Lucy says, "Charlie Brown, you blockhead, I love the world. It's the people I can't stand." That won't work. Love is encouragement. Encouragement for yourself and others. Remember to encourage people. It starts a healthy flow. NO ONE EVER DIED FROM AN OVERDOSE OF ENCOURAGEMENT.

Relax Every Day!
Picture Health!

Exercise!
Participate!
Believe in Something Beyond Yourself!
Set Goals!
Have Fun!
Be Positive!
Eat Right!
Choose Love and Encouragement!
Hang on to Your Hope!

Above all, I am certain that hope is healthy. Do not be afraid to hope. Hope ties it all together.

Final note: Read about health. Ask questions of your doctors. Believe in yourself, and become an active participant in your own wellness and wholeness.

Here's to your health!

Patient Guide

The sense of helplessness that many cancer patients feel is the most debilitating effect of our society's attitude toward the disease. Many people who must face the diagnosis feel that they can only lie back and suffer whatever cancer dishes out. Some even refuse medical treatment, believing that passive acceptance or active refusal are their only options.

That popular idea is not true. You can fight cancer by becoming an active participant in your treatment program. By applying the principles described in this guide, you will become a working partner with the rest of your medical team to fight the disease in your body.

These principles sound so commonplace that they may not appear to be therapeutic. They are so worn with use that you might overlook them as you search for support and comfort. It is their very usefulness that has made them seem commonplace, for they are part of every wise man's life.

- People are healthier if they practice regular relaxation. Relaxation helps people who are sick to "go with the flow" and to put their energy into recovery.

- Focusing on health and envisioning healing helps people prevent and fight off disease. Our dreams have a way of coming true. Dreams of wholeness give us the power to heal.

• Active participation in our own health care allows us to cease feeling victimized and to begin working toward health.

• A clear faith in a power greater than ourselves benefits our health. A clear life philosophy or a religious faith deepens our experience and helps us to stay well.

• Laughter and fun are not trivial distractions. They are as much a part of life's whole as are tears and sorrow. You'll live longer and be healthier if you enjoy life.

• Positive attitudes and thoughts empower us to attain health.

• A high-fiber, low-fat, regulated diet is healthy. If we eat right, we live longer and healthier.

• Love and encouragement buoy us up. We were made to love one another. We need to help others along the way and to seek out people who do the same for us.

• Hope and a sense of purpose pull us onward. If we have something to live for, we may live longer, and our lives will certainly be more worth living. Hope ties everything else together.

No one questions the seriousness of the disease: cancer. We who work with cancer patients know that your body will need all the energy you can summon to fight this invader. If you learn how to reduce tension, fear, depression, and other energy-draining emotions, however, your body will marshall its forces more effectively and focus them on fighting the cancer.

The purpose of the program described in this booklet is to help you reduce the need to deal with stress and negative emotions, to help you recover vitality and hope, and to assist you in learning techniques that will enable you to cooperate with whatever treatment you are receiving. We believe that this will help you to make the best possible use of your body's natural resources.

We also want to help you improve the quality of your life. It isn't only that we want you to live more fully whatever time you have left, even though that is a worthy goal for all of us. We also believe that, as the quality of your life improves, your enjoyment of life will increase, your desire to live will intensify, and you will use up less energy coping with despair and anxiety. The result will be not only a fuller life, but a longer life, and, in some cases, the restoration of health.

How much this program will help you is largely up to you. It will not be enough merely to read the guide. You must make the commitment to practice what you learn with all the dedication of the most devoted religionists in the world or with the discipline of a serious athlete. It is not enough to know. You must also do!

The principles recommended here can work to make your life better and longer. The major question may be whether you want improved health enough to really work at this program, one day at a time. If you do, then you can expect positive results in your life. We are asking you to approach these instructions with devotion and determination.

This plan is "An Adjunct Treatment Program for Cancer Patients." It is called "adjunct" because it supplements whatever regular or conventional treatment, such as radiation or chemotherapy, you are receiving. *This program is not a substitute for other treatments.* All of your doctors, nurses, technicians, psychologists, clergy, and others are working with you as a team, fighting the cancer that has invaded your body.

This program is called "treatment," but it might just as accurately be called "education" or "training." We want to help you aid your medical treatment through education and training.

There are four strands in this program: relaxation, visualization, new ways of thinking, and exercise. You will be on your own in applying what you learn. We cannot motivate you to do what you are unwilling to do, but remember that we are asking you to work as if your life depended on what you do. In fact, it may.

1. *Relaxation training:* The first element of the program is a technique that, with practice, will help you relax. We begin here because this tool will enable you to control stress and tension. All of us experience tension in some degree and can profit from learning to release it, but the purpose here is more than easing present tensions. We want to help you learn a technique, a tool, that you can call upon whenever you experience tension of any kind. A relaxed body is freer to function normally. Relaxation also reduces pain. And people are more open to learning other new techniques when they are relaxed.

The relaxation technique described here is an effective one, well-tested in the laboratory and clinical practice. It involves sitting in a quiet place and practicing the relaxation of your muscles in groups, beginning with your facial muscles and going through the other muscles all the way to your feet.

It is common knowledge that stress reduces the body's resistance to disease. Research suggests that excessive stress increases certain hormones that retard the immune system. It stands to reason that, if stress reduces resistance, it also impedes recovery from disease. If you learn to relax, your body will be free to fight the cancer.

One woman in our pilot study found that relaxation relieved the nausea she had experienced before, during, and after her chemotherapy treatments. In *her* case, nausea was caused more by tension resulting from fear than by the chemotherapy drugs. Other positive effects will undoubtedly result from the use of relaxation techniques.

Relaxation is something you can achieve. It is something you can do on your own, as well, a place where you can begin to participate in your own health. Make an audio tape of the following instructions, or ask someone to read them slowly for you as you respond, step by step. Use the tape at least twice a day until you have learned the instructions. The relaxation process should last about ten to twelve minutes.

- Find a quiet, comfortable place.

- Sit or lie down and close your eyes.

- Take a deep breath and hold it for about five seconds, then slowly release it.

- Breathe normally for a moment and say to yourself, "When I inhale, I breathe in relaxation. When I exhale, I breathe out tension."

- Breathe in relaxation and health, breathe out tension and impurities.

- Now take another deep breath. Hold it for about five seconds and slowly release it.

- Let your body relax. Think of it as a bag filled with sand. Let your muscles fall apart.

- Take your time, and become conscious of the muscles in your forehead. Briefly raise your eyebrows up toward the top of your head, and let them fall.

- Let the relaxation begin to flow down your face.

- Think of the muscles around your eyes. Squint briefly, then let your eyes relax.

- Move your attention to the muscles in your jaws. Clench your jaws briefly, then let them relax.

- Focus your attention on your neck. Move your head from side to side, then let it tilt forward if you are sitting, or fall back if you are lying down.

- Think of your shoulders. Shrug them up toward your ears and let them fall.

- Feel the relaxation that started in your forehead flow down over your face and into your neck and through your shoulders into your upper arms.

- Tighten the muscles in your upper arms briefly, then let them relax.

- Think of your lower arms. Make fists, then let your fingers straighten until the relaxation seems to drain through them.

- Roll your shoulders forward to stretch the muscles in your back. Let the muscles relax.

- Think of your chest. Push it out briefly, then let it relax.

- Push your stomach toward your back, then let it out. Imagine that your stomach is like a pile of soft rubber bands.

- Arch your lower back forward, then let it relax.

- Tighten your hip muscles, then let them relax.

- Think of the muscles in your upper legs. Tighten them briefly, then let them relax.

- Think of your lower legs. Lift your toes toward your knees, and then push them down. Now relax.

- Let every muscle in your body just fall apart as you take a deep breath and slowly release it.

- Now you can open your eyes at your own pace and go about doing whatever you want to do.

• If you wish, you are ready now to practice visualization.

When you have mastered this exercise, you probably will be able to induce a relaxed state by simply closing your eyes and taking a deep breath or by imagining a relaxing scene. Use this skill when you are receiving treatments. It can also help you sleep more restfully.

2. *Positive visualization:* The process of visualizing a goal is not new. Scientists have used it to solve problems. Baseball players have improved their pitching accuracy and raised their batting averages by imagining themselves succeeding. The idea of fighting cancer with this method, however, is relatively new.

Imagination and visualization can accomplish truly amazing results. People who see themselves running activate the muscles in their legs; laboratory instruments have measured these contractions. In other experiments, human beings have altered body processes such as brain wave patterns and blood pressure, by means of mental imagery. Young men in another study dramatically improved their performance in darts and basketball free-throws, solely by means of mental practice.

Visualizing skills are applicable in any area of life. You can use them to fight cancer. The idea is to imagine your own body and your medical treatment effectively fighting, controlling, and even destroying the cancer in your body. Create a mental picture of your white blood corpuscles attacking and killing cancer cells, your radiation therapy effectively hitting its targets, and your chemotherapy doing its job efficiently. See your own body's defense system consciously cooperating with your treatments to destroy cancer in your body.

The evidence indicates that positive visualization helps. Even if it did nothing else, it would at least help you to believe that the destruction of cancer cells is possi-

ble. To see it is to be able to believe it! This belief increases your hope. Hope displaces despair and thus helps
you relax and use your energy for healing. Every time you
practice your relaxation exercise, use your imagination to
see the very thing you want actually happening. This discipline could be compared to a game of "let's pretend," but
it is not a game, and it is not just pretending. It is visualizing a potential reality.

Not only will visualization help raise your hope, it
will deepen your relaxation and make it easier for your
whole system to cooperate in fighting cancer. Remember,
once again, that the technique will benefit you only if you
do it, at least twice a day.

3. *Changing your thinking:* "Cognitive restructuring"
is a fancy name for changing the way you think. We will
employ a variety of thinking techniques to help you deal
with fears, frustrations, pain, depression, and expectations. This is another thing you can do yourself, a skill
you can apply in any area of your life.

Basically you are learning to rethink your fundamental beliefs about yourself and the world. At one point in
your life, you learned to think and believe as you do. Your
reactions are not automatic by nature; they are learned. As
children, we hear something, repeat it in our thoughts,
and silently file it away for future reference. We learn
through repetition. Using the same process by which you
learned your ideas in the first place, you can substitute
more realistic, helpful, and positive ways to think and react.

Some of the things we learned as children are false
and may, in fact, harm us. We may have learned to believe crippling things about ourselves. We often become
unwitting fulfillers of our own negative prophecies.

As an example of how our thinking affects the course
of our lives, imagine two people who have lost their jobs.
The first person reacts to the experience by becoming de-

pressed and suicidal. The second may be disappointed, but nevertheless vigorously pursues a new job. The experience affects them differently because they believe different things about the situation and talk to themselves in different ways.

"Oh, my God, I've lost my job," the first person says. "I'm a failure. I'll never get another job. My life is not worth living." Such thinking naturally leads to depression.

The second person sees things differently. "Well, I lost my job. That's bad, but it is not the end. I can work, and I'll start looking tomorrow." This sort of thinking leads not to depression, but to a new job!

Something happens to you. You talk to yourself about it, and discuss your beliefs with yourself. Then you react according to your internal discussion. The same kind of process occurs when your doctor tells you that you have cancer. You begin to go over your beliefs. You may say, "Oh, God, I've got cancer. There is no hope for me. I'm going to die right away, and I probably will have a lot of pain and disfigurement." If you believe and say that, the result is despair, depression, and panic.

You may honestly believe these statements, but they are not necessarily true. Suppose you say something different to yourself: "I have cancer. That's bad, but it isn't the end of the world. As long as I can fight, there is hope. I will do everything I can to overcome this thing. Life is fickle anyway, and anyone may die at any time. My problem is to make my life as full and meaningful and healthy as possible. Now let me see. What can I do now to help myself?"

If you react to your bad news with such beliefs, you are likely to feel a lot better. The point is that if you learn to change your beliefs and the way you discuss them with yourself, you can change the way you feel. Emotions can be controlled.

We are not proposing that you put on a happy face

and pretend to be stoic and brave. In fact, expressing the emotions you really do feel is important to your recovery. We are not urging you to embrace positive ideas that are untrue, just because they're positive. That kind of pretense won't do you any good. But you can change the prophecies of doom and other beliefs you have that are negative and false, because they damage you.

The process is simple. First, become aware of your present beliefs about yourself, the world, and other people. Pull into your mind the thoughts that make you frightened, tense, and depressed. Part of becoming conscious of your emotions is being completely honest and open about them. Are you angry? Do you hold some resentment? Do you feel guilty? Are you afraid? Are there other feelings you have never dealt with honestly? Face these things.

When you identify an emotion that has to do with cancer, take a private inventory to find out what beliefs generated that emotion. What are you saying internally? Whatever it is, write down that belief. It is a hypothesis about your situation. Now that you have it identified, examine it. Do a little research. Check with your physicians to see whether your information is correct. If not, then write down the new information.

Begin to make two lists. Write any negative original belief you may have about yourself and your disease on the left side of a page. Across from each old belief, on the right side of the page, revise the belief; state the original idea in a more positive way.

Now learn the list on the right side of the page. Say these statements aloud. Memorize the new beliefs. Use them as often as you can. Say them to your friends and relatives. Whenever you think the old thought, replace it with the new one. Use the old only as a stimulus for the new. You are now consciously changing your thoughts. As you do so, the emotions, fears, frustrations, depressions, and general misery associated with the old ideas will change too. Teach yourself new ideas. They will change your emotions.

Any kind of emotion can be dealt with in this way, for feelings are usually the result of our beliefs. Examine the thoughts behind it, write down the thoughts or beliefs, check them to see if they are really valid, then rewrite them in more positive words.

The lists that follow will help you get started, if you want to change your fears of cancer or death, your depression, your sense of helplessness.

If you suffer from depression, keep a list for a week of all the depressing thoughts you notice. You may hear yourself saying these things aloud, or you may be aware of the fact that you are saying them to yourself. Write the depressing thoughts on the left side of the page. Then, on the right side of the page, opposite each negative thought, write a more positive or encouraging way to interpret the same topic, and write that statement on the right side of the page. Examples are listed below.

Depressive Thought	*Positive Thought*
No one cares what happens to me.	Some people care what happens to me. *I* care!
Nothing good ever happens to me.	Some good things happen to me, and a lot more good can happen.
I'm sick and I'm going to die.	Everyone is going to die and none of us knows when. But I can live whatever life I have as fully as possible.
People make me miserable.	I have been making myself miserable, and I can stop it.

If you have trouble thinking of positive statements,

ask a trusted friend to help you verbalize the positive or encouraging statements.

An additional skill will help you deal with other difficult emotions. Learn to formulate statements that you can say to yourself. Fear, for example, is a universal human experience. It cannot be denied away, but it can be confronted. First, become aware of your fears and the experiences that produce them. When you have identified your fear, use the following guide for help in confronting and coping with it. These are statements you might repeat to yourself. You may want to add other statements of your own. Some of the statements that follow will help you when you anticipate something that makes you fearful, others when you are experiencing a present fear.

- When you feel fear or know you are facing a fear-producing event:
  "I'll describe my fear or what I have to do."
  "I can think of a plan to deal with it."
  "I'll think about what I can do. That's better than getting anxious."
  "I'm not going to make negative statements to myself."
  "I'll think through this rationally."
  "I won't worry. Worry doesn't help."
  "I will face this thing and I'll make it!"

- When the fear is present or a "fear event" is taking place:
  "I'll 'psych' myself up. I can meet this challenge."
  "I'll reason it away."
  "One step at a time I can handle this situation."
  "I won't concentrate on fear. I'll think of what I can do."
  "I'll relax. I'm in control. I'll take a deep breath."
  "I'll label my fear from 0 to 10 and watch it change."
  "I won't try to eliminate fear totally; just keep it manageable."
  "I'll pause now and focus on the present."

- After you have coped with your fear, reinforce
yourself:
"It worked; I did it!"
"My ideas—they are the problem. When I control
them I do all right."
"Wait until I tell my friends about this!"

Pain is another universal human experience. All of us
have felt pain in the past and will certainly experience
more. You can help yourself to deal with pain by preparing yourself for it. Practice the following statements, or
devise statements of your own and practice them.

- Preparing for pain:
"What is it that I have to do?"
"I can develop a plan to deal with this."
"I'll think about what I can do."
"I won't worry. Worry doesn't help."
"There are a lot of strategies I can call upon."

- Confronting and handling pain:
"I can meet this challenge."
"One step at a time, I can handle this situation."
"I'll stop thinking of pain and think instead about
what I can do."
"I'll relax, take a deep breath, and use one of my
strategies."
"I'll relax. I'm in control. Now I'll breathe deeply."
"This pain just reminds me to use my new skills."

- Coping with feelings at critical moments:
"When the pain comes, I'll pause and keep focusing
on what I can do."
"I am thinking, 'What is it I have to do?'"
"I won't try to eliminate pain totally, just keep it
under control."
"If pain mounts, I can switch strategies and stay in
control."

• When you feel relief from pain:
"Good, I did it."
"I handled that pretty well."
"I knew I could do it"
"Wait until I tell my friends about this."

Pain may generate stress. If you have pain, you need a strategy for coping with it. Select one of the following coping strategies, and use it as part of your plan.

• Attention diversion: Focus your attention on things other than your pain. Do mental arithmetic, for example. Study the pattern in your clothing. Count ceiling tiles. Find any activity that requires your concentration and focus on that activity.

• Somatization: Focus your attention on your bodily processes or sensations. For example, observe and analyze the feelings in your body that may result from the pain you are experiencing.

• Imagery manipulations: Change or transform the experience of pain by means of imagery. Use your imagination to create a fantasy that is incompatible with pain. Imagine that you are doing something you enjoy, like lying on a beach in the sun. Or imaginatively transform your pain into a fantasy that includes pain but minimizes the sensation. For example, fantasize that you are feeling cold or numbness, rather than pain. Or use your imagination to transform the context of your pain. Fantasize an experience that includes pain, but change the context. Imagine, for example, that you are feeling a pulled muscle as you cross the goal line for a touchdown, or a gunshot wound you have received while in the line of duty for your country.

If none of these strategies feels comfortable or natural, develop your own method.

4. *Exercise:* The fourth strand in this training program is more than a fad in America. It is an essential element in any person's health program. Proper exercise keeps our blood circulating freely and helps us breathe easier. It seems that our bodies are made for exercise. Research has indicated for seventy years that active bodies more effectively resist and fight cancer. Tissues from fatigued muscles in mice have been shown to retard cancer.

We are not suggesting that you overdo exercise, of course. Use your own good judgment to tailor the following guidelines into an exercise routine that fits your own needs.

- Set aside one hour at least three times per week.

- If you have not been exercising, use light exercise like walking and simple movement of your arms.

- Increase your exercise gradually and use as a guideline your ability to converse while doing it. As long as you can maintain a conversation, you are probably within safe limits.

- Choose your own exercises, but make them light enough to continue for the full hour.

- Carry on normal activities as much as you can.

When people are sick, they are usually told to rest, but too much rest can, in some cases, be detrimental. Remember that you are responsible for your own program. You can do it. Only you can do it.

Both relaxation and exercise relieve stress. Here are several additional ideas that may also be helpful, and you may come up with others.

- Learn to ask the right questions. When you meet a situation that has produced anger, frustration, or depression in the past, take a deep breath and ask yourself, "How do I want to respond to this situation?"

• Learn to put things in perspective with important questions like: "Who says?" "So what?" Or the big one, "Is this worth dying for?" You never get good answers until you ask the right questions.

• Have fun! Consciously choose to have as much fun as you possibly can. If you can make a situation laughable, do it. Laughter can heal.

• Keep variety in your life. Try new things, eat new foods, go to new places, try new hobbies, or just change your daily schedule. Variety reduces stress. If you carry a suitcase in one hand, that arm and hand become stressed. Change hands!

• Practice your religious faith. If your faith is positive, it will relieve stress. Take the responsibility for finding and expressing your own faith or philosophy. It is your right.

Exercise, relax, have fun, spice your life with variety, and find your own meaningful faith. Whatever their circumstances, people who do these things find that their lives improve. That is true for young people, old people, people in good health, and people with cancer.

You need not abandon your life and accept whatever happens, like a sacrificial lamb. You can take charge of yourself, in ways this guide suggests. If you do that, you will undergo the trials of medical treatment with higher spirits than you ever thought you could muster. As an active member of the team, you will make the most of the treatment plan. And you will come through it with a new pride in your own personal power.

All good wishes to you on your journey!

Suggested Reading

Cousins, Norman. *Anatomy of an Illness.* New York: Bantam Books, 1979.

Garrison, Judith Garrett, and Scott Sheperd. *Cancer and Hope, Charting a Survival Course.* Minneapolis: CompCare Publishers, 1989.

Hargrove, Anne C. *Getting Better, Conversations with Myself and Other Friends While Healing from Breast Cancer.* Minneapolis, CompCare Publishers, 1988.

LeShan, Lawrence. *You Can Fight for Your Life.* New York: M. Evans and Company, 1977.

Little, Bill L. *This Will Drive You Sane.* Minneapolis: CompCare Publishers, 1977.

Robbins, Anthony. *Unlimited Power.* New York: Fawcett-Columbine, 1986.

Selye, Hans. *The Stress of Life.* New York: McGraw-Hill, 1956.

Siegel, Bernie S. *Love, Medicine and Miracles.* New York: Harper and Row, 1986.

Simonton, Carl O., and Stephanie Simonton. *Getting Well Again.* Los Angeles: J. P. Tarcher, 1978.

About the Author

Bill L. Little, a native of Gideon, Missouri, holds a B.A. from East Texas Baptist College, a Th.M. from Midwestern Baptist Theological Seminary, an M.S. from Southern Illinois University, and a Ph.D. from Washington University.

For over thirty years, he has been pastor of Christ Memorial Baptist Church in St. Louis. For over twenty, he has been a professional therapist. Since 1977 he has been known to a wide radio audience for his on-the-air counseling over station KMOX, St. Louis. He has been team psychologist for two baseball teams—the St. Louis Cardinals from 1980-82, and the Seattle Mariners from 1983-87—using visualization techniques to help improve sports performance. He has taught at Washington University, University of Missouri in St. Louis, and Missouri Baptist College, and has conducted conferences on alcoholism marriage and family relations, stress communications, management and motivation.

He is the author of *This Will Drive You Sane* (CompCare) and several magazine articles.